DEADLY DISEASES AND EPIDEMICS

STREPTOCOCCUS (GROUP A)

Second Edition

Anthrax, Second Edition

Antibiotic-Resistant Bacteria

Avian Flu

Botulism, Second Edition

Campylobacteriosis

Cervical Cancer

Chicken Pox

Cholera, Second Edition

Dengue Fever and Other Hemorrhagic Viruses

Diphtheria

Ebola

Encephalitis

Escherichia coli Infections, Second Edition

Gonorrhea

Hantavirus Pulmonary Syndrome

Helicobacter pylori

Hepatitis

Herpes

HIV/AIDS

Infectious Diseases of the Mouth

Infectious Fungi

Influenza, Second Edition

Legionnaires' Disease

Leprosy

Lung Cancer

Lyme Disease

Mad Cow Disease

Malaria, Second Edition

Meningitis, Second Edition

Mononucleosis, Second Edition

Pelvic Inflammatory Disease

Plague, Second Edition

Polio, Second Edition

Prostate Cancer

Rabies

Rocky Mountain Spotted Fever

Rubella and Rubeola

Salmonella

SARS, Second Edition

Smallpox

Staphylococcus aureus Infections

Streptococcus (Group A), Second Edition

Streptococcus (Group B)

Syphilis, Second Edition

Tetanus

Toxic Shock Syndrome

Trypanosomiasis

Tuberculosis

Tularemia

Typhoid Fever

West Nile Virus, Second Edition

Whooping Cough

Yellow Fever

DEADLY DISEASES AND EPIDEMICS

STREPTOCOCCUS (GROUP A)

Second Edition

Tara C. Smith, Ph.D.

CONSULTING EDITOR:
Hilary Babcock, M.D., M.P.H.,
Infectious Diseases Division,
Washington University School of Medicine,
Medical Director of Occupational Health (Infectious Diseases),
Barnes-Jewish Hospital and St. Louis Children's Hospital

FOREWORD BY
David Heymann
World Health Organization

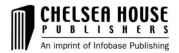

CHELSEA HOUSE
PUBLISHERS
An imprint of Infobase Publishing

Streptococcus (Group A), Second Edition

Copyright © 2010 by Infobase Publishing

Chelsea House
An imprint of Infobase Publishing
132 West 31st Street
New York NY 10001

Library of Congress Cataloging-in-Publication Data

Smith, Tara C., 1976–
  Streptococcus (group A) / Tara C. Smith ; consulting editor, Hilary Babcock ; foreword by David L. Heymann. — 2nd ed.
    p. cm. — (Deadly diseases and epidemics)
  Includes bibliographical references and index.
  ISBN-13: 978-1-60413-251-9 (hardcover : alk. paper)
  ISBN-10: 1-60413-251-5 (hardcover : alk. paper) 1. Streptococcal infections. 2. Streptococcus. 3. Necrotizing fasciitis. I. Babcock, Hilary. II. Title. III. Series.

  QR201.S7S63 2010
  616.9'298—dc22
                          2009048579

Text design by Terry Mallon
Illustrations by Dale Williams
Cover design by Takeshi Takahashi
Composition by Mary Susan Ryan-Flynn
Cover printed by Bang Printing, Brainerd, MN
Book printed and bound by Bang Printing, Brainerd, MN
Date printed: June 2010
Printed in the United States of America

10 9 8 7 6 5 4 3 2 1

This book is printed on acid-free paper.

Table of Contents

Foreword

Communicable diseases kill and cause long-term disability. The microbial agents that cause them are dynamic, changeable, and resilient: They are responsible for more than 14 million deaths each year, mainly in developing countries.

Approximately 46 percent of all deaths in the developing world are due to communicable diseases, and almost 90 percent of these deaths are from AIDS, tuberculosis, malaria, and acute diarrheal and respiratory infections of children. In addition to causing great human suffering, these high-mortality communicable diseases have become major obstacles to economic development. They are a challenge to control either because of the lack of effective vaccines, or because the drugs that are used to treat them are becoming less effective because of antimicrobial drug resistance.

Millions of people, especially those who are poor and living in developing countries, are also at risk from disabling communicable diseases such as polio, leprosy, lymphatic filariasis, and onchocerciasis. In addition to human suffering and permanent disability, these communicable diseases create an economic burden—both on the workforce that handicapped persons are unable to join, and on their families and society, upon which they must often depend for economic support.

Finally, the entire world is at risk of the unexpected communicable diseases, those that are called emerging or reemerging infections. Infection is often unpredictable because risk factors for transmission are not understood, or because it often results from organisms that cross the species barrier from animals to humans. The cause is often viral, such as Ebola and Marburg hemorrhagic fevers and severe acute respiratory syndrome (SARS). In addition to causing human suffering and death, these infections place health workers at great risk and are costly to economies. Infections such as Bovine Spongiform Encephalopathy (BSE) and the associated new human variant of Creutzfeldt-Jakob disease (vCJD) in Europe, and avian influenza A (H5N1) in Asia, are reminders of the seriousness of emerging and reemerging infections. In addition, many of these infections have the potential to cause pandemics, which are a constant threat to our economies and public health security.

Science has given us vaccines and anti-infective drugs that have helped keep infectious diseases under control. Nothing demonstrates the effectiveness of vaccines better than the successful eradication of smallpox, the decrease in polio as the eradication program continues, and the decrease in measles when routine immunization programs are supplemented by mass vaccination campaigns.

Likewise, the effectiveness of anti-infective drugs is clearly demonstrated through prolonged life or better health in those infected with viral diseases such as AIDS, parasitic infections such as malaria, and bacterial infections such as tuberculosis and pneumococcal pneumonia.

But current research and development is not filling the pipeline for new anti-infective drugs as rapidly as resistance is developing, nor is vaccine development providing vaccines for some of the most common and lethal communicable diseases. At the same time, providing people with access to existing anti-infective drugs, vaccines, and goods such as condoms or bed nets—necessary for the control of communicable diseases in many developing countries—remains a great challenge.

Education, experimentation, and the discoveries that grow from them are the tools needed to combat high mortality infectious diseases, diseases that cause disability, or emerging and reemerging infectious diseases. At the same time, partnerships between developing and industrialized countries can overcome many of the challenges of access to goods and technologies. This book may inspire its readers to set out on the path of drug and vaccine development, or on the path to discovering better public health technologies by applying our current understanding of the human genome and those of various infectious agents. Readers may likewise be inspired to help ensure wider access to those protective goods and technologies. Such inspiration, with pragmatic action, will keep us on the winning side of the struggle against communicable diseases.

David L. Heymann
Assistant Director General
Health Security and Environment
Representative of the Director General for Polio Eradication
World Health Organization
Geneva, Switzerland

1

One Bacterium, Many Different Diseases

At the age of 53, Jim Henson, creator of the Muppets and several children's television shows, appeared to be healthy. In May 1990, however, Henson complained of fatigue and a sore throat. He assumed he had a case of influenza. Despite getting rest, his symptoms worsened. He was having difficulty breathing by the time his wife, Jane, took him to New York Hospital. Although doctors immediately began to give him intravenous antibiotics, the infection had already progressed too far to respond to treatment. About 20 hours later, Jim Henson died as his kidneys and heart ceased to function. His death was caused by streptococcal toxic shock syndrome, a disease caused by group A streptococci.

The group A beta-hemolytic streptococcus (GABHS; species name, *Streptococcus pyogenes*) is a species of bacteria that can cause a wide variety of diseases. Some of these diseases may be superficial (nonlethal) diseases, such as **pharyngitis** (strep throat) and **impetigo** (a skin disease). However, infections caused by some strains (isolates that are identical at the genetic level) of this type of bacterium can also cause diseases with a high fatality rate, such as **necrotizing fasciitis (NF)** and **streptococcal toxic shock syndrome (STSS)**. In addition, diseases caused by these bacteria do not necessarily stop affecting the person when the infection is eliminated. Indeed, some diseases only begin to manifest symptoms days or weeks after the bacteria have been cleared from the body. These delayed diseases, called **postinfection sequelae**, are most often due to an aberrant immune response by the host. Some postin-

DISEASES CAUSED BY
STREPTOCOCCUS PYOGENES

Strep throat

Scarlet fever

Impetigo

Erysipelas

Cellulitis

Necrotizing fasciitis

Wound infections

Toxic shock syndrome

Puerperal fever

Rheumatic fever

Glomerulonephritis

fection sequelae include **glomerulonephritis** (a disease of the kidneys), **rheumatic fever**, and **rheumatic heart disease**. The group A streptococcus is also able to cause **scarlet fever**, which is a rash caused by toxins produced by the bacteria during a throat infection; and **puerperal fever**, which is a postpartum infection of the blood that was, at one time, a leading cause of mortality among women who had recently given birth.

One aspect of the biology of group A streptococci that is both interesting about this group of bacteria, as well as frustrating to those who study it, is that the **epidemiology** (study of disease patterns) of the organisms has changed over time. For example, during some points in history, infection with a group A streptococci almost always resulted in only a mild disease, such as pharyngitis. However, at other times, group

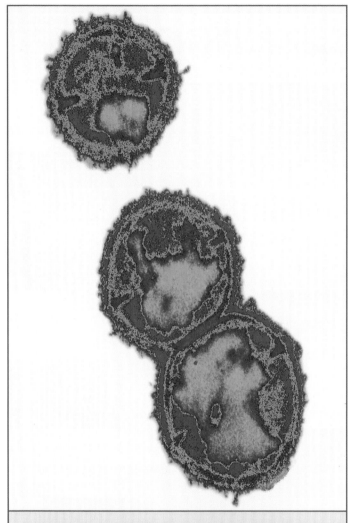

Figure 1.1 This electron micrograph shows individual cells of group A streptococci, magnified almost 30,000 times. (© Dr. George Chapman/Visuals Unlimited, Inc.)

A streptococci were the causative agents of deadly epidemics, which could result in the death of every child in a family. Most recently, a resurgence of severe diseases caused by GABHS has been observed. In the 1980s, after being viewed for decades as a relatively harmless pathogen affecting mainly children, deadly diseases caused by GABHS made an alarming return in developed countries. This change in epidemiology has led the **Centers for Disease Control and Prevention** (CDC) to classify group A streptococci as **reemerging pathogens.**

PUERPERAL FEVER

Infections caused by the group A streptococcus cause some of the oldest scourges of humankind. Indeed, one of the earliest well-described diseases, puerperal fever, is caused by infection with these bacteria. Puerperal fever is an infection that may occur in women shortly after childbirth (and because of this, it is also referred to as "childbed fever"). This infection was characterized as long ago as 1500 B.C. by the ancient Hindus, even though they had no concept at that time of the **germ theory of disease** (the idea that microorganisms—including bacteria, viruses, and fungi—are responsible for causing contagious diseases). The famous ancient Greek physician Hippocrates, in his treatise on diseases of women, also described the disease around 400 B.C. At that time, it was believed that the disease was caused by the suppression of the **lochia** (the vaginal discharge that occurs in the weeks after childbirth). This suppression, in turn, was thought to cause an imbalance in the body **humors** (the fluids in the body, such as blood and bile).

Although childbed fever was an ancient illness, it remained a relatively rare cause of death until "advances" in obstetrics led to an increase in gynecological operations and an increase in births in hospitals. Pregnant women were more likely to have invasive procedures performed on them in a hospital, to be crowded in a room with several patients, and to be exposed to contaminated bed linens and medical instruments. These situations led to an increase in the **mortality** (rate of death) from puerperal fever.

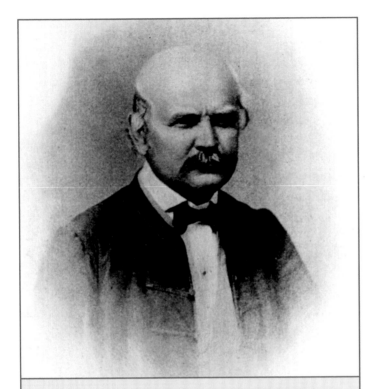

Figure 1.2 Ignaz Semmelweis (1818–1865) played a key role in the reduction of mortality due to group A streptococcal infections in the late nineteenth century. He was one of the first advocates of handwashing and used a chlorinated solution to reduce transmission of infectious agents between patients. (National Library of Medicine)

DISCOVERY OF STREPTOCOCCUS PYOGENES

In the late eighteenth century, some British physicians suspected that contagion caused puerperal fever. Cleanliness and chlorination of the hospital wards were recommended to combat the disease, resulting in mild success. A Hungarian-born physician, Ignaz Semmelweis, carried these practices further and made great strides in determining the cause of puerperal fever.

Semmelweis was a lecturer in the department of obstetrics in a Vienna hospital where medical students were trained.

Between 1841 and 1843 the mortality rate caused by puerperal fever in the division where medical students treated patients was 16% (8 out of 50 women died of puerperal fever). However, in the division of the hospital where midwives performed deliveries, the mortality rate was only about 2% (1 out of 50 women died of puerperal fever). Semmelweis also observed that very few women who gave birth at home died of puerperal fever. The more he thought about it, the more convinced Semmelweis became that the cause of childbed fever could be found by closely investigating the practices of the medical students and comparing them to those of the midwives.

Unfortunately, it took a tragedy to lead Semmelweis to the cause of the disease. In 1847 Semmelweis's friend and colleague, Jakob Kolletschka, died of a wound incurred during a **postmortem** dissection. At the autopsy, Semmelweis noticed that the **pathology** he found in Kolletschka's body was the same as the changes observed in the bodies of women who had died of puerperal fever. He quickly realized the implications of his findings: The medical students performed autopsies, whereas the midwives did not. The students, as a result, brought contagious material directly from the autopsy room to the delivery room; at that time, handwashing was not used as a way to prevent the spread of disease.

That same year Semmelweis began to require students to wash their hands in a chlorinated solution before they could enter the maternity ward. The results were immediate and dramatic. Mortality from puerperal fever in the medical students' division fell from 11.4% in 1846 to approximately 3% at the end of 1847.

Semmelweis's ideas were scoffed at by other physicians of his day. He was not reappointed to his position in the Allgemenines Krankenhaus (a university in Vienna, Austria). Instead, he took a position as an obstetric physician at another hospital, in Budapest, in 1849, where he again instituted his handwashing practice and reduced the mortality rate from puerperal fever to less than 1%. In 1865 Semmelweis was committed to a psychiatric clinic in Vienna. Within a few weeks, he died, disgraced and alone.

HIPPOCRATES, THE "FATHER OF MEDICINE"

Hippocrates (460 B.C.–377? B.C.), known as the "father of medicine," was born in Greece. Hippocrates's most important contribution to medicine was his refusal to believe that the actions of gods could be used to explain illness. Instead, he stressed the importance of observation and science to understand disease. He believed that illness occurred because of an imbalance of one of the body's four "humors," or fluids: blood, black bile, yellow bile, and phlegm. If the body contained either too much or too little of any of these fluids, illness resulted. Hippocrates also emphasized the importance of fresh air, exercise, and healthy eating to assist the body's healing mechanisms. Although his ideas on the body's humors were accepted for many centuries after his death, his ideas about exercise and healthy eating were, for the most part, forgotten until recent times.

Students of Hippocrates had to follow a strict code of ethics that governed their behavior as physicians. Doctors still take the Hippocratic oath today, an oath that has changed very little since Hippocrates's day.

Ironically, the same disease he had fought against throughout his entire professional career proved to be the death of him: He succumbed to **septicemia** (bacteria in the bloodstream) from a cut he sustained on his finger during an operation he performed on a newborn baby before he was committed.

In the years after his death, the practices Semmelweis had advocated to reduce deaths from puerperal fever gradually came to be instituted in hospitals around the world. However, the reason the methods worked was unknown. The germ theory of disease was being developed and refined around this

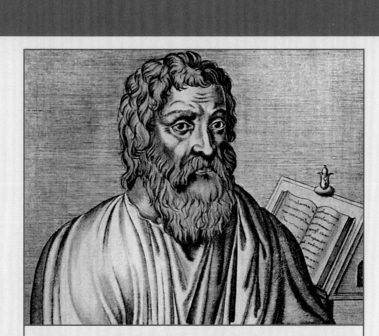

Figure 1.3 Hippocrates (460 B.C. –377?B.C.), one of the world's earliest physicians, is also often credited as the father of medicine. He developed a set of ethical guidelines for physicians, called the "Hippocratic oath," which is still followed today. (National Library of Medicine)

time by scientists such as Robert Koch, working in Germany, and Louis Pasteur, a French scientist. Pasteur in particular was instrumental in recognizing that the group A streptococcus was the cause of puerperal fever. He had been observing cases and taking samples of patients' blood in an effort to determine the cause (which he believed to be an infectious agent). During a visit to Pitié Hospital, Pasteur was able to obtain blood and pus from a woman dying of puerperal fever. In it, he saw a familiar germ; Pasteur was now certain he had discovered the bacterium responsible for puerperal fever.

In May 1879 Pasteur attended a meeting of the Académie de Médecine. He listened to a presentation on puerperal fever by a noted gynecologist, who discounted the idea that "germs" were the cause of this disease. Rather, he spoke of **miasmas**— "bad airs" that were believed at that time to be a significant cause of disease. Pasteur interrupted the speaker, stating, "What causes the epidemic is none of these things; it is the physician and his helpers who transport the microbe from a sick woman to a healthy woman." Pasteur then proceeded to the blackboard, and drew a picture of the bacteria he had found in his samples from the case at Pitié Hospital and elsewhere: bacteria that looked remarkably like a string of pearls.

Stunned, the gynecologist invited Pasteur to visit his practice in the Lariboisié hospital the very next day. Samples were taken from women who were ill with puerperal fever. As Pasteur had predicted, the samples all contained bacteria in the shape of chains of pearls, which were christened "*Streptococcus pyogenes*" (group A streptococcus) in 1884. This discovery led the way for a more scientific application of **aseptic** practices, because scientists knew that the chlorinated handwashing solution worked by killing the bacteria present on the hands.

A DEADLY SORE THROAT

Streptococcal toxic shock syndrome (STSS) is a severe invasive disease caused by *Streptococcus pyogenes* that emerged in the 1990s. In the early 1990s this syndrome was just beginning to increase in **incidence** (the number of cases of the disease that have been newly diagnosed during a given year). Until this disease caused the untimely death of Jim Henson, however, the general public was largely unaware of it.

The syndrome generally occurs when group A streptococci gain access to the blood, often through a breach in the skin. When they enter the bloodstream, the bacteria produce a protein known as a **superantigen**. This protein (of which there are several varieties) overwhelms the body's defenses, leading to

shock (a decrease in blood pressure, leading to a lack of blood flow to the organs) and organ failure, which causes death in approximately 30% of individuals who develop the disease.

FLESH-EATING DISEASE

In the early 1970s another type of severe infection surfaced in North America and Europe. This infection was named necrotizing fasciitis (NF) because of the **necrosis** (tissue death) that causes inflammation of the **fascia** (tissue underlying the skin). NF is similar to STSS in that it is an invasive streptococcal disease that can quickly lead to death. Because of the gruesome nature of the disease and its clinical manifestations, the media dubbed NF the "flesh-eating disease."

The death of a beloved public figure, coupled with the arrival of a frightening new manifestation of group A streptococcal disease that received a great amount of media attention, led to a resurgence of interest in these bacteria.

SUMMARY

Even before it was discovered or named, the group A streptococcus had been a scourge to mankind. Though some diseases it caused in the past (for example, puerperal fever) have all but disappeared, others (such as STSS) have surfaced to take their place. These bacteria remain a major threat today. Epidemics caused by this bacterium have waxed and waned, and the severity of the illnesses it causes has varied over time. However, one thing has remained constant: the presence of these bacteria in the human population. The diseases caused by group A streptococci, the microbial and host factors responsible for the development of illness, and the medical treatments used to restore the patient to health will be examined in the following chapters.

2

Diagnosis and Treatment of the Group A Streptococcus

The name *Streptococcus pyogenes* (group A streptococci, or GABHS), coined in 1884, literally means "fever-causing twisted chain of berries," due to their appearance when viewed under a microscope. These bacteria belong to a group of organisms that are called ***gram-positive*** *cocci*. This term describes characteristics of both the bacteria's shape and general cell wall structure. **Coccus** (plural, *cocci*) refers to the round shape of the bacterium when viewed under a microscope. Because of the **Gram stain**, the bacteria will also appear to be purple in color. This stain helps micro-biologists distinguish the bacteria from gram-negative bacteria and from other related gram-positive organisms, such as *Staphylococcus aureus*, which do not grow in chains. Other means used to identify and character-ize GABHS will be discussed later in this chapter.

TRANSMISSION OF THE GROUP A STREPTOCOCCUS

Group A streptococci live only in humans; they are not found anywhere else in nature. In humans, they are generally found in the **nasopharyngeal** passages (the nose and the throat), and occasionally on the skin. Although these bacteria can survive for short times on inanimate objects, such as doorknobs and countertops, and may occasionally be transmitted via these means, GABHS are most commonly transmitted through direct person-to-person contact. They can be spread this way through the air via fluid droplets leaving the nose or throat when someone sneezes or speaks, or via shared eating utensils, such as forks, spoons, or drinking glasses. Because these bacteria are most commonly spread from person to person, the peak incidence of infection with these bacteria occurs during the winter months, when people are most often indoors. School-age children have the highest incidence of infection with these bacteria.

Because GABHS are transmitted directly through the air or indirectly via objects that harbor bacteria, the best way to prevent infection is through frequent handwashing and avoidance of sick contacts. If a family member or friend is infected, it is

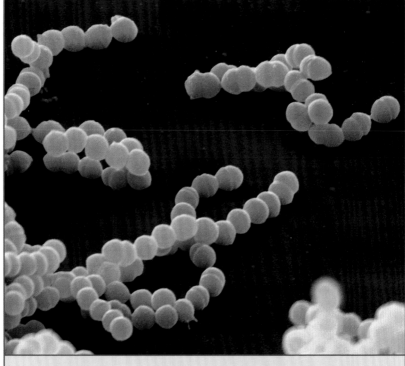

Figure 2.1 Electron micrograph of group A streptococci. Note the typical "chain of pearls" form taken by the bacteria. (© Eye of Science/Photo Researchers, Inc.)

best to avoid sharing any utensils and to make sure all glasses and silverware are washed carefully in hot, soapy water.

DIAGNOSIS

Streptococcal infections, primarily streptococcal pharyngitis, cost billions of dollars every year in the form of doctors' visits, medication, and lost workdays in the United States. Acute pharyngitis is one of the most frequent illnesses for which pediatricians and other primary care physicians are consulted. Although GABHS remains the leading bacterial cause for this acute disease, it is still the causative agent for only a minority of all pharyngitis cases. Indeed, most cases of pharyngitis are caused by various viruses, against which antibiotic treatment is useless.

The most common test to determine whether GABHS is the cause of sore throat is to culture the bacteria on a **blood agar plate**. This growth media consists of agar mixed with sheep's blood, solidified in a petri dish. The test, called a throat culture, consists of swabbing the throat (or skin pustules, in the case of suspected streptococcal impetigo) with a sterile cotton swab. The swab is then wiped onto the surface of the blood agar plate, and the plate is allowed to incubate overnight at 98.6°F (37°C). The following day, the plate will be examined to see if evidence of hemolysis (breaking open red blood cells) is present around the bacterial colonies (if there are any) on the blood agar plate. Colonies of GABHS will be whitish in color, with a clear zone around the colony where the bacterial **hemolysins** have lysed the sheep red blood cells. If additional chemical tests confirm that the bacteria are indeed *Streptococcus pyogenes*, an antibiotic regimen can be started immediately.

One limitation to throat culture is that the bacteria must be grown overnight to have a sufficient quantity of bacteria to observe, increasing the amount of time before the patient receives treatment. However, in recent years, this technology has been either replaced or enhanced by the introduction of rapid antigen detection testing (RADT). This test also begins with a swab of the patient's throat; however, it employs a chemical reaction to look for the presence of particular antigens present on the bacteria. The RADT can produce a result in as little as 10 minutes; therefore, treatment can begin sooner, reducing the amount of time the patient is contagious.

Unfortunately, RADT also has limitations. It may be less sensitive than the traditional throat culture, particularly if the bacteria in the throat are present at low concentrations. This means that if a person is infected with a low number of the bacteria, the rapid test may falsely say that the patient is not infected (this is called a "false negative" result). It may also produce a "false positive" result, indicating the presence of bacteria that are not actually there. However, with the tests available today, this is unlikely. Finally, it is more costly than a throat culture. Often, a throat culture is performed as a precaution, in order to confirm the results of the RADT.

PUTTING THE "A" IN GROUP A STREPTOCOCCI

Once a clinical microbiologist observes colonies that appear to be GABHS growing on blood agar plates, further tests can be done to positively identify the bacteria. The first goal is to confirm the identification of group A streptococci. After colonies have grown on blood agar plates, a Gram stain can be used as the next step in identification. For this procedure, bacterial colonies are removed from the blood agar plate and spread on a glass slide, where they are heated quickly to fix the bacteria to the slide. The bacteria are then stained with a reagent called crystal violet. The bacteria take up this dye and appear purple in color. Iodine is then used to "fix" this dye within the bacterial cells, which are then treated with a decolorizing agent, such as ethanol. In gram-positive organisms, the thick cell wall prevents the decolorizing agent from entering the cell and removing the violet dye; therefore, these cells will remain purple. In gram-negative bacteria, the thick cell wall is not present; therefore, the bacteria lose their color when the decoloring agent is applied. To visualize the gram-negative cells, a stain called safranin is

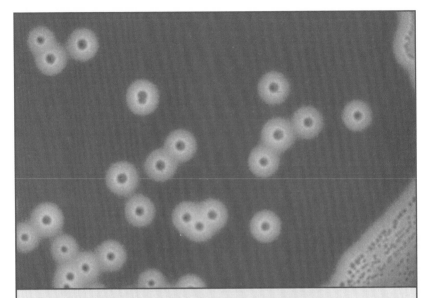

Figure 2.2 Group A streptococci causing hemolysis on sheep blood agar plate. The clear zones around the bacterial colonies are the result of the lysis of red blood cells within the agar, which occurs when the bacteria release hemolysins. (© Dr. Gladden Willis/Visuals Unlimited, Inc.)

used. The end results are purple for gram-positive bacteria and pink-colored (safranin-stained) for gram-negative bacteria. These slides can then be viewed under a microscope, and cells can be differentiated based on their color and shape. Recall that GABHS are gram-positive cocci (spheres) that grow in chains.

Once it is deemed likely that GABHS are present based on the tests described above, the bacteria can be grouped according to features of this species. In order to understand how this is done, it is helpful first to understand some definitions used by clinical microbiologists. First, a **strain** of a bacterium is one that has certain defined characteristics—whether they are at the level of the **genotype** (genetic code) or the **phenotype** (appearance and behavior of the bacterium). In contrast, an **isolate** of a bacterium is similar to an individual human; it is unique. All individual isolates of the bacterium can be grouped into strains. If we think of isolates as individuals, we can think of strains as families: Though they can be taken from different geographic locations (for example, an identical strain may be found in a patient in New York and another in California), they are all closely related. The combination of all known strains makes up the bacterial species.

People's ability to understand the epidemiology of *Streptococcus pyogenes* has been enhanced largely because of the pioneering work of Rebecca Lancefield. Lancefield developed a way to distinguish *Streptococcus pyogenes* from other related but different species of streptococcus. She based this typing on a particular carbohydrate antigen (bacterial surface molecule) that is common to all strains of *Streptococcus pyogenes*, but absent in other streptococcal species. This antigen was designated the "A" antigen (it is for this reason that *Streptococcus pyogenes* is also referred to as "group A streptococcus").

SEROTYPE AND THE M PROTEIN

Lancefield also examined what made each strain of GABHS different not only from other species, but from other strains within the species. Lancefield determined that the M protein (a protein on the cell surface of GABHS) conferred **serotype** (group of similar strains that will all be recognized by a host immune response) specificity to each isolate. In her animal studies, she determined that mice infected with one serotype isolate were protected from further disease caused by that identical serotype. In most cases, however, the mice were not protected from disease caused by isolates of a different serotype. This discovery led to the development of **antisera** (serums that contain antibodies) specific to each known serotype of group A streptococci. These antisera have been used by researchers worldwide to type their collections of GABHS isolates. More than 100 different serotypes of GABHS have been identified. Individual isolates are generally identified by their serotype; for example, isolates of serotype 1, 3, and 18 are most commonly isolated from cases of invasive disease today.

REBECCA LANCEFIELD, MICROBIOLOGY PIONEER

Rebecca Lancefield (née Craighill, 1895–1981) was a woman in a field dominated by men. Like many women in that position, she defied stereotypes and forged a new path. She received her doctorate in bacteriology from Columbia University in 1925 for her work on streptococci. Upon completion of her degree, Lancefield accepted a position at the Rockefeller Institute to work on hemolytic streptococci, which, at that time, had recently been implicated in the development of rheumatic fever. However, research into the different species of streptococci was still in a relative state of chaos. Lancefield's work contributed much to the field. In 1928 she published a series of papers in the *Journal of Experimental Medicine* describing the M protein and the group-specific polysaccharide. She continued work in this research for many decades.

In 1943, Lancefield was elected president of the Society of American Bacteriologists, the second woman to become president of that society. However, because of restrictions placed on travel during World War II, she was unable to preside over a national meeting. She later served as president of the American Association of Immunologists (1961), becoming the first woman to serve in that office. In 1970, she was elected to membership in the National Academy of Sciences, becoming only the 11th woman to achieve that honor. Currently, the name "Lancefield" is associated throughout the world with the typing of species and strains of streptococci.[1]

Although this identification method was reliable, it suffered from several inherent difficulties. First, the antisera were quite expensive to make, store, and transport. Second, there would inevitably be isolates that did not react with any of the known antisera; these were simply designated "untypeable" isolates. In some areas, such as Australia, there often were more "untypeable" isolates than isolates that could be serotyped with the available antisera. Third, the method depended on being able to extract sufficient quantities of the M protein from the surface of the bacteria. Because some isolates would stop producing M protein after a culture was made in the laboratory, extracting adequate quantities was difficult. With the advent of molecular biology, the typing of M proteins using antisera has been replaced with a molecular typing method.

Using the latter method, the *emm* gene (which encodes the M protein) is directly **sequenced** (that is, the nucleotide — DNA — sequence of the gene is determined). The gene can then be compared to known *emm* gene sequences specific to each serotype. This molecular typing method is less expensive than the antisera technique and is easier to reproduce between different laboratories. Additionally, since strains that were "untypeable" using antisera were now able to be assigned a "type" based on the genetic sequence of the *emm* gene, even more variability has been discovered within GABHS. There are now more than 120 known molecular types of this bacterium.

TREATMENT

Most patients who have been diagnosed with a streptococcal infection should begin antibiotic therapy immediately, with an appropriate antimicrobial agent. A number of different antibiotics have been shown to be effective in treating streptococcal infections. These include penicillin (as well as similar antibiotics, including ampicillin and amoxicillin), numerous cephalosporins and macrolide drugs, and clindamycin. Penicillin remains the drug of choice because of its low cost, **efficacy**, safety, and narrow spectrum (meaning it kills only a few particular species of bacteria). Young children are frequently given amoxicillin instead of penicillin because the former is thought to work slightly better. However, recent research has shown that a class of antibiotics called cephalosporins work better to treat streptococcal infections. This represents an improvement over penicillin/amoxicillin treatment in two ways: Cephalosporins are more effective at treating the infection, and they are also given over a shorter period of time (typically 3–5 days, versus a 10-day regimen of penicillin/amoxicillin).[2]

In some cases antibiotics do not kill all of the infecting bacteria. This may be because the dose of antibiotics was too small, because the patient did not finish his or her entire prescription, or because the bacteria already harbored **resistance** to the prescribed antibiotic. In some cases only a small proportion of the bacteria was resistant when the patient began his or her course of antibiotics. The antibiotics will kill the susceptible bacteria. This will then allow the antibiotic-resistant bacteria to multiply, since there are more nutrients available after the antibiotic-susceptible bacteria are killed off. In some cases a new antibiotic can be used to treat the infection. In other cases the bacteria are resistant to all known antibiotics, and the infection is essentially untreatable.

Fortunately, antimicrobial resistance has not been a significant issue in the treatment of group A streptococcal infections in the United States. In fact, despite the fact that penicillin has been used for years in treating group A streptococcal infections, no clinical isolate of GABHS has been identified anywhere in the world that shows resistance to the drug. However, in many areas of the world, relatively high levels of resistance to some classes of antibiotics, including macrolides, have been documented. In the United States, a decade ago, less than 5% of clinical isolates were resistant to erythromycin. A recent study has shown that, for isolates collected between 2003 and 2006, almost 15% were resistant to erythromycin, and 1.4% were resistant to another commonly used drug to treat GABHS infections, clindamycin.[3] This rapid increase in antibiotic resistance is a concern, and a reminder that people need to be vigilant about not overusing antibiotics. Patients should always complete their prescribed course of antibiotics to prevent resistant bacteria from surviving and causing a second infection. Currently, most oral antibiotics are prescribed for a 10-day period and are highly effective at clearing the bacteria from the throat.

3

Superficial Infections: Streptococcal Pharyngitis and Impetigo

Carlos awoke Monday morning with a scratchy throat, feeling slightly warm. He took his temperature and found it was a bit elevated at 100° Fahrenheit. He felt the lymph nodes on the side of his neck and could tell they were somewhat swollen. "Uh oh," he thought. "Bad sign." He dug out a flashlight from underneath his kitchen cupboard and headed into the bathroom. Looking into the mirror above the bathroom sink, he said "ah" and stuck out his tongue as far as he could, shining the flashlight into his throat—which looked red. Carlos had streptococcal pharyngitis ("strep throat") twice already in the past year. Each time, even though he went to his doctor and received an antibiotic prescription as soon as he noticed symptoms, he still felt ill and tired for several days, and because he was contagious, had to miss several days of his work as a waiter each time he was sick.

Carlos called his physician and scheduled an appointment later in the morning. The nurse checked his throat and temperature, and took a swab of the back of this throat and put it on a little circle on the strep "rapid test," which would quickly tell her whether Streptococcus pyogenes was present in his throat. (She also streaked this swab on an agar plate, where bacteria could grow). She returned in five minutes: the test had come back positive. His physician returned and wrote Carlos a prescription for amoxicillin, an antibiotic, and recommended lots of rest and fluids. Carlos would also have to stay home from work for two days while the antibiotics worked to reduce the number of bacteria present in his throat, so that he would not spread the infection to friends and coworkers.

A disease that causes a minor or localized infection is generally termed a **superficial disease.** Generally, these diseases are minor in scope and self-limited. This means that they will often clear up on their own, without treatment, and will rarely become serious or life-threatening. Superficial diseases caused by the group A streptococcus (GAS) include a skin infection called impetigo and pharyngitis, an infection of the epithelium of the throat. Over 10 million superficial GAS infections occur annually in the United States alone.

STREPTOCOCCAL PHARYNGITIS

Pharyngitis is the medical term for a painful inflammation of the throat (pharynx); in other words, "strep throat." Direct costs associated with pharyngitis in the United States have been estimated to be $1 billion annually, making it one of the most costly infectious diseases in the world today. Most often, pharyngitis is caused by a virus, which is not treatable with antibiotics. Strains of GABHS are found to be the cause of pharyngitis in approximately 15% of cases of sore throats in children. When pharyngitis is caused by this bacterium, it is most often accompanied by a fever above 101°F (38°C). In addition, the child may experience chills, body aches, a decrease in appetite, nausea, abdominal pain, and vomiting. The tonsils at the back of the throat may appear swollen and red, and are often dotted with white or yellowish spots of **pus.** Swallowing is often difficult because of the condition of the throat.

The symptoms of streptococcal pharyngitis vary slightly when infants contract this infection. Like older children, they may eat poorly; but infants often exhibit a runny nose and frequently have sores and crusting around the nostrils. Streptococcal pharyngitis rarely infects infants.

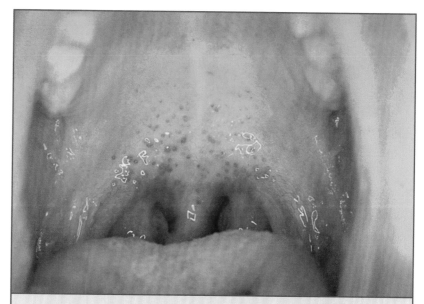

Figure 3.1 This is the throat of a child who has an active strepto-coccal infection. Note the characteristic redness and swelling of the tonsils. (Centers for Disease Control and Prevention)

The **incubation period** (time between the initial exposure to the bacteria and the development of the disease) for GABHS is generally between 2 and 7 days. After that, the fever often will last approximately 3–5 days, with the sore throat diminishing during that time or shortly afterward. If left untreated, the infected person will be **contagious** (able to transmit the bacteria to others) during almost the entire duration from the time the bacteria begin multiplication in the host until the end of symptoms. However, two days after antibiotics are administered, a person is no longer contagious.

There are also cases where persons (particularly children) can carry GAS in their nasopharynx (the upper part of the pharynx, connected to the nasal passages), but do not have any symptoms of strep throat. These people are referred to as **asymptomatic carriers**. Although they show no outward signs

FOODBORNE OUTBREAK OF GROUP A STREPTOCOCCUS

Large epidemics of pharyngitis caused by *S. pyogenes* are relatively rare; foodborne epidemics even more so. However, *S. pyogenes* can contaminate food, and can infect individuals who eat the food. In June 2006 an outbreak of streptococcal throat infections occurred among employees in an office building in Denmark. Out of approximately 1,000 people working in the building, at least 140 became ill with sore throat. Investigations showed that the only common exposure all sick employees had was that they had all eaten in the office cafeteria. Most cases had eaten either from the salad bar or chosen the warm vegetarian dish, which was a hot pasta dish.

Food inspectors investigated conditions at the cafeteria, taking swabs from cooking utensils, food products, and food service workers. One worker was found to have a wound on his thumb; he was also involved in the preparation of the pasta dish implicated in the outbreak. He was found to be a carrier of *S. pyogenes*, and analysis of the bacteria from his throat showed that they matched isolates taken from other office building employees who had become ill.

Inspectors also noticed that refrigeration procedures in the cafeteria appeared inadequate. Leftovers of the hot pasta were stored in a large plastic bin and placed in the refrigerator. The large, tightly filled bin meant that the pasta took longer than expected to cool to refrigeration temperatures; therefore, any bacteria present in the pasta could have multiplied on the pasta even while in the refrigerator. When this leftover pasta was served the next day, this could have infected additional employees. However, because none of the food products remained by the time the investigation was carried out, this could not be proven. This report represented the largest food-borne outbreak of *S. pyogenes* in Europe in 30 years, highlighting the importance of thinking about food as a vehicle for transmission in outbreaks of this pathogen.[1]

of illness, they still are able to transmit the bacteria to others. Between 10 and 20% of school-age children are thought to be asymptomatic carriers of GABHS.

In addition, although throat infections with GABHS are rarely serious in and of themselves, researchers have shown that many of these pharyngeal strains have the potential to cause serious invasive disease. Thus, both people with active streptococcal pharyngitis, as well as **healthy** (or asymptomatic) **carriers**, can serve as a source of deadly bacteria.

In rare cases, strep throat infections that are not treated with antibiotics (or cases that are treated, but fail to kill all the bacteria) can lead to more severe diseases, even after the sore throat appears to be healed. These severe diseases include rheumatic fever, an illness that can lead to further complications, such as heart disease and arthritis. Another condition, glomerulonephritis, a kidney disease, can follow pharyngitis by approximately 2–3 weeks.

Large-scale outbreaks of streptococcal pharyngitis are relatively rare. Generally, transmission is limited to close contacts, such as family members or a group of children in a day-care center. However, larger epidemics do occur occasionally. One such outbreak took place in December 1999 in an Australian prison where 72 inmates came down with tonsillopharyngitis, thought to be spread by infected kitchen workers. A similar outbreak occurred in Denmark in June 2006.

IMPETIGO

Impetigo is a skin infection that can be caused by either group A streptococci or by *Staphylococcus aureus.* In the United States and much of Europe, impetigo usually affects children (preschool or school age) and is most common in the summer months (when other skin conditions such as poison ivy, insect bites, and eczema may make children more likely to contract the disease).

Impetigo caused by GABHS generally begins as small skin blisters. When these blisters burst, small patches of skin are

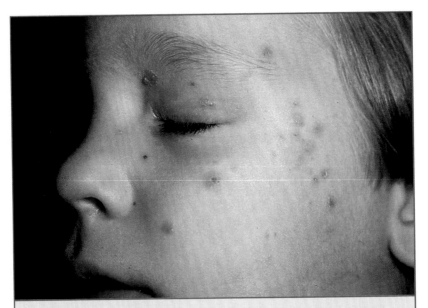

Figure 3.2 This child's face shows the most common sign of streptococcal impetigo. The small skin blisters will become yellow and crusted as they heal. Impetigo most often affects the skin of the face, mouth, and nose. (© Dr. Ken Greer/Visuals Unlimited, Inc.)

revealed. These patches are red in color and may produce fluid. As the infection heals, a yellowish crust forms over the area.

Although impetigo can affect any area of the body, the skin around the mouth and nose are most often affected. Just as with other skin diseases, impetigo may be itchy. Scratching the blisters may cause them to burst and bacteria on the fingers and beneath the fingernails can then spread the disease to other areas of the body or transmit it to others. Although direct contact is the most common way impetigo is spread, it can also be spread by touching infected clothing, linens, and towels. As with streptococcal pharyngitis, the patient generally ceases to be contagious approximately 48 hours after beginning an antibiotic regimen. Again, frequent handwashing remains the best way to prevent this disease.

Although impetigo remains only a minor health problem in the United States, it is a major problem in aboriginal communities in areas of Australia, where up to 70% of children can be infected. One reason that underlies this problem is the fact that **scabies**, a skin condition caused by mites, is a common disease and causes breaks in the skin that allow group A streptococci easy access to the underlying tissue. These high rates of infection also take a toll on the population because of an increased prevalence of invasive GAS infections that may follow skin infections, as well as a high rate of post-infection sequelae, such as glomerulonephritis and rheumatic fever. Rates of rheumatic fever in Australia are among the highest anywhere in the world.

4

Scarlet Fever

Julie bolted up out of bed, hearing the pattering of her six-year-old daughter Aurora's feet approaching down the hallway. Aurora told her mother that she didn't feel good. Julie felt Aurora's head; she was sweaty and burning up with fever. Julie carried Aurora into the bathroom and fished some fever-reducing medicine out of the medicine cabinet. She placed a wet washcloth on Aurora's forehead to mop up some of the sweat and cool her off a bit while she placed a thermometer in her ear to take her temperature. Aurora's shirt was also soaked with sweat, so Julie pulled it off and reached around to grab a clean shirt out of the laundry pile, when she noticed a rash on Aurora's belly and chest, stopping just short of her neck. After putting Aurora back to bed with a glass of water, Julie called the pediatrician, who advised her to bring Aurora in for an examination.

The pediatrician checked out Aurora's rash, and looked at Aurora's red, swollen throat and her strawberry-red tongue. She took a swab of Aurora's throat for confirmation, and Julie was surprised at the probable diagnosis: scarlet fever. The pediatrician explained that it was relatively rare, but that it occasionally occurred, especially in children. She gave Aurora a reassuring pat on the head and explained the antibiotic regimen to Julie, and sent them both home for some rest and chicken soup.

In recent history, the most famous and most dreaded form of streptococcal infection was scarlet fever. Simply hearing the name of this disease, and knowing that it was present in the community, was enough to strike fear into the hearts of people who lived 150 years ago in the United States and Europe. This disease, even when it was not deadly, caused large amounts of suffering to those infected. In the worst cases, all of a family's children died within a week or two.

From ancient times up until the early twentieth century, scarlet fever was a common condition among children. In fact, the disease was so common in the United States that it was central to the popular children's tale *The Velveteen Rabbit* (1922), in which the central character contracts scarlet fever, and must have his belongings—including his cherished velveteen rabbit—destroyed to prevent transmission or recurrence of the disease.

Luckily, scarlet fever is much less common today in developed countries than it was when Williams's story was published. In fact, many doctors practicing in the United States today have never seen a case of scarlet fever firsthand. However, having doctors who are unfamiliar with the disease also puts us at a disadvantage, should a scarlet fever epidemic ever again sweep the nation.

SYMPTOMS

Most often, this infection is localized in the throat (**tonsillopharyngitis**). Rarely, scarlet fever occurs after the skin infection, impetigo. Children with scarlet fever develop chills, body aches, loss of appetite, nausea, and vomiting; these symptoms may occur at the same time as or shortly following the onset of pharyngitis. When the scarlet fever rash emerges, it generally appears as a severe, itchy sunburn with tiny bumps. After first becoming visible on the neck and face, it spreads to the chest and back, later spreading to the arms and the remainder of the body. Though the rash initially consists of separate bumps, these bumps tend to merge together, giving the entire torso a red appearance. Generally, the rash begins to fade by about the sixth day; as with sunburn, the skin may peel afterward.

Although the rash is the most obvious symptom, and the one from which the name of the disease is derived, other symptoms help confirm the diagnosis of scarlet fever. As mentioned, sore throat is often present, as well as a fever (above 101°F, or 38.3°C) and swollen glands. The tonsils and back of the throat may be covered with a whitish coating and may appear red and

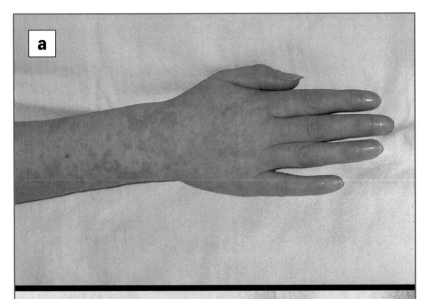

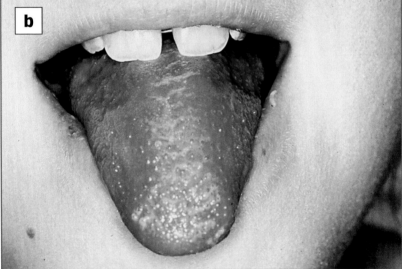

Figure 4.1 The hand and arm of this individual show the typical scarlet fever rash (a). Often, the spots merge to become a solid redness on the skin, and will peel like a sunburn as the rash heals. Another common symptom of scarlet fever is the development of "strawberry tongue" (b). (© Mediscan/ Science VU/Visuals Unlimited, Inc.)

WAS THE PLAGUE OF ATHENS CAUSED BY GROUP A STREPTOCOCCI?

The plague of Athens remains one of the great medical mysteries in history. First breaking out in the year 430 B.C., the plague killed approximately one-third of those infected, and quickened the end of the Golden Age of Greece. The plague spread quickly within the walls of Athens. The city was at war with Sparta at the time and was housing as many as 200,000 extra people, who had fled their homes for the relative safety of the walled city. Thus, the wartime chaos and crowding made the inhabitants of Athens particularly vulnerable to an epidemic of infectious disease.

Thucydides (471–400 B.C.), a historian and plague survivor, described the disease in his *History of the Peloponnesian War*, Book II, Chapter 49:

[1] That year then is admitted to have been otherwise unprecedentedly free from sickness; and such few cases as occurred, all determined in this.

[2] As a rule, however, there was no ostensible cause; but people in good health were all of a sudden attacked by violent heats in the head, and redness and inflammation in the eyes, the inward parts, such as the throat or tongue, becoming bloody and emitting an unnatural and fetid breath.

[3] These symptoms were followed by sneezing and hoarseness, after which the pain soon reached the chest, and produced a hard cough. When it fixed in the stomach, it upset it; and discharges of bile of every kind named by physicians ensued, accompanied by very great distress.

(continues)

(continued)

[4] In most cases also an ineffectual retching followed, producing violent spasms, which in some cases ceased soon after, in others much later.

[5] Externally the body was not very hot to the touch, nor pale in its appearance, but reddish, livid, and breaking out into small pustules and ulcers. But internally it burned so that the patient could not bear to have on him clothing or linen even of the very lightest description; or indeed to be otherwise than stark naked. What they would have liked best would have been to throw themselves into cold water; as indeed was done by some of the neglected sick, who plunged into the rain-tanks in their agonies of unquenchable thirst; though it made no difference whether they drank little or much.

[6] Besides this, the miserable feeling of not being able to rest or sleep never ceased to torment them. The body meanwhile did not waste away so long as the distemper was at its height, but held out to a marvel against its ravages; so that when they succumbed, as in most cases, on the seventh or eighth day to the internal inflammation, they had still some strength in them. But if they passed this stage, and the disease descended further into the bowels, inducing a violent ulceration there accompanied by severe diarrhea, this brought on a weakness which was generally fatal.

[7] For the disorder first settled in the head, ran its course from thence through the whole of the body, and even where it did not prove mortal, it still left its mark on the extremities.

[8] For it settled in the privy parts, the fingers and the toes, and many escaped with the loss of these, some too with that of their eyes. Others again were seized with an entire loss

of memory on their first recovery, and did not know either themselves or their friends.

Thucydides goes on to say that those who recovered from the disease were not stricken by it again. Additionally, much like the Black Plague that followed a millennium later, bodies piled up too quickly to be attended to in an orderly manner. Many people were eventually buried in mass graves.

Although the causative agent of the plague of Athens is still uncertain, as many as 30 different diseases have been suggested. These include malaria, Ebola, *Yersinia pestis* (the agent that causes bubonic plague), yellow fever, influenza, typhus, and *Streptococcus pyogenes.* The evidence for the latter comes from the description of the nature of the rash and throat involvement, the general weakness, the rapidity of disease onset and death, and the neurological symptoms that were present upon recovery. Additionally, necrotizing fasciitis can also lead to the loss of extremities.

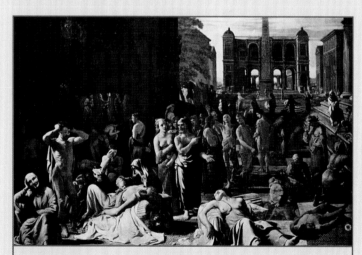

Figure 4.2 This painting by French painter Nicholas Poussin (1594–1665) depicts the plague in Greece during the fifth century B.C. (© Michael Sweerts/The Bridgeman Art Library/ Getty Images)

swollen. In some cases, they may be dotted with whitish or yellowish specks of pus. Early in the infection, the tongue also may have a whitish coating and turn red ("strawberry tongue") as its surface begins to peel.

Today, scarlet fever is rarely fatal. When death does result, it can be due to a number of different reasons. These include septic shock, which is a response by the body's immune system that can lead to generalized organ failure. Causes of death can also include more specific bacterial attacks on individual organs, leading to failure. These most often include the heart and kidneys. **Meningitis** or **encephalitis** (swelling of the brain) caused by the bacteria may also result in death. The nature of the rash also **predisposes** a person to secondary bacterial infections (that is—infections that take advantage of the breaks in the skin caused by the scarlet fever rash). This is infrequently a cause of death.

WHAT CAUSES SCARLET FEVER?

Some strains of group A streptococcus produce proteins, called **toxins**, that cause a rash in those who are sensitive to the toxin. In GABHS, these toxins are referred to as **Streptococcal Pyrogenic Exotoxins**, or **SPEs**, for short. The particular strain of bacteria may possess more than one type of SPE. Currently, it is not clear which SPE (or combination of SPEs) is most important in the development of scarlet fever.

HISTORICAL PERSPECTIVE

The earliest case definition of scarlet fever is a matter of debate. Some researchers believe that descriptions of a disease that match scarlet fever date back almost 2,500 years, to ancient Greece and Hippocrates. Others believe the first conclusive diagnosis is found in writings by Arab physicians from the tenth century. It is generally agreed that the first sufficiently detailed paper identifying scarlet fever as a disease distinct from other rashes appears in 1553. In that paper the Italian physician

Giovanni Filippo Ingrassia describes the disease and refers to it as "rossalia." The term **febris scarlatina** appears in a 1676 publication by the British physician, Thomas Sydenham.

Historical data suggest at least three epidemiologic phases for scarlet fever. In the first, which appears to have begun in ancient times and lasted until the late eighteenth century, scarlet fever was either **endemic** (always present in the population) or occurred in relatively benign outbreaks separated by long intervals. In the second phase (c. 1825–1885), scarlet fever suddenly began to recur in cyclic and often highly fatal urban epidemics. In the third phase (c. 1885 to the present), scarlet fever began to manifest as a milder disease in developed countries, with fatalities becoming quite rare by the middle of the twentieth century.

During Sydenham's life (1624–1689), and for more than a century afterward, both laypeople and physicians considered scarlet fever a relatively mild childhood disease. Although several European cities experienced fatal epidemics of the disease, these were often short-lived, and it does not appear that they were widespread.

In the early nineteenth century, however, the clinical presentation of the disease appears to have changed for the worse. Lethal epidemics were seen in Tours, France, in 1824; in Dublin, Ireland, in 1831; and in Augusta, Georgia, United States, during 1832–1833. Similarly, in Great Britain, the fatality rate from scarlet fever increased from between 1 and 2% to more than 15% in 1834.

From 1840 until 1883 scarlet fever became the most common infectious childhood disease to result in death in most of the major metropolitan centers of Europe and the United States, with fatality rates that reached or exceeded 30% in some areas. In some documented cases, several children in the same family died from the disease in a matter of weeks. In one case a British family abandoned their house after four of their five children died from scarlet fever. After a three-month absence and after disinfecting the house with carbolic acid, they returned with their sole remaining child, only to have the child die of scarlet fever less than two weeks later. In this case, the possibility of a servant serving as an asymptomatic carrier was suggested retrospectively as the possible source of the bacteria. Scarlet fever pandemics of this and other eras also had a profound effect on history.

In both England and the United States, mortality from scarlet fever began to decrease around the year 1883. By the

ROLE OF SCARLET FEVER IN THE LIVES OF PROMINENT PEOPLE

Scarlet fever was a major cause of childhood mortality in the late nineteenth century. At the time, some infectious diseases affected those of lower socioeconomic classes because of poor nutrition and crowded living conditions. Scarlet fever, however, killed indiscriminately, taking the lives of the rich and poor alike. As a result, many notable persons living during the nineteenth century were affected by a personal loss because of this dread disease.

Charles Darwin (1809–1882), the father of evolutionary theory, lost two of his children to scarlet fever. The first, his beloved daughter Annie, died at the age of 10 in 1851 (two of Darwin's other daughters, also infected, recovered from this bout). At Annie's memorial service, Darwin stated,

> We have lost the joy of the Household, and the solace of our old age:—she must have known how we loved her; oh that she could now know how deeply, how tenderly we do still & shall ever love her dear joyous face. Blessings on her.

In July 1858, Darwin also lost his 18-month-old son, Charles Waring, to scarlet fever.

middle of the twentieth century, the mortality rate from scarlet fever again fell to around 1%. The cause of this decline in virulence remains unknown. Alan Katz and David Morens, in a 1992 paper, put forth one potential explanation:

> One possibility is that such virulent strains were of comparatively lower transmissibility than other strains competing for the same ecological niches. In the early and mid-19th century in Europe and the United States,

It is believed that a bout of scarlet fever at the age of 19 months caused Helen Keller (1880–1968) to lose her senses of vision and hearing. However, through the efforts of a caring teacher, Annie Sullivan, Helen learned to use sign language and read Braille. She eventually graduated from Radcliffe College with honors. In later years she became an advisor and active fund-raiser for the American Foundation of the Blind. She worked tirelessly throughout her life to show that people with disabilities could contribute to society in many ways.

The world's first billionaire and the founder of Standard Oil, John D. Rockefeller (1839–1937), donated money from his personal fortune to the American Foundation of the Blind. He also assisted Keller in her fund-raising efforts. Rockefeller, like many Americans at the time, had experienced the death of a loved one from scarlet fever. In Rockefeller's case, it was his three-year-old grandson, John Rockefeller McCormick, who died of scarlet fever. In 1901 Rockefeller founded the Rockefeller Institute for Medical Research, the first organization in the United States devoted solely to medical research. In 1965 this became Rockefeller University. It remains a leader in biomedical research today, and continues to investigate various aspects of the biology of the group A streptococcus.

such factors as industrialization, urbanization, rural and urban population shifts, and crowding might have allowed such otherwise poorly transmissible but virulent strains to gain a foothold in urban areas. At the turn of the 20th century, decreased crowding; the practice of isolating infected persons in homes, schools, and hospitals; advances in sanitation and hygiene; and rising immunity among the population over the 60-year prevalence of such virulent strains could have combined to limit their urban circulation, thereby delaying and limiting spillover to rural areas and to developing countries.

Scarlet fever still remains a threat today, particularly in developing countries. However, nowhere is it now as severe a disease as it was during the frightening years in the middle of the nineteenth century.

RECENT OUTBREAKS OF SCARLET FEVER

Though scarlet fever is nowhere near the scourge it was during the Victorian Era, it still remains a disease of concern. Recent outbreaks of scarlet fever have been reported among children in Mexican day-care centers and orphanages. Of greatest concern is the finding that the outbreak strain isolated from the infected day-care children was resistant to **erythromycin**, a drug commonly used to treat streptococcal infections.

Although scarlet fever is no longer a leading killer of children, group A streptococci remain the cause of other serious, and sometimes lethal, diseases.

5

Resurgence of an Old Pathogen: Invasive Streptococcal Diseases

Bridget woke up with a strange pain in her left side, running from her shoulder down her side, and down her arm. She'd been feeling tired and sick for the last few days and figured she was suffering from the flu, but this new pain didn't seem to be flu-related at all. Despite taking pain relievers, the soreness and tenderness worsened. By the next morning, Bridget was in horrible pain and couldn't get out of bed, and asked her husband to take her to the doctor.

Bridget spent the morning at the urgent care center, where they thought she may have pneumonia. However, they noticed that her blood pressure was very low and fever was very high, and decided to send her to the emergency room for further evaluation.

At the ER, they found that Bridget's white blood cell count was very high—a sign of an infection. Finally, after over 12 hours of X-rays, blood tests, and other examinations, her physician told her he had determined what was wrong with her, and that she was in for the fight of her life. He told Bridget that she had necrotizing fasciitis, or "the flesh-eating disease," and that they would need to take her to surgery immediately; she didn't even have time to call her children or other family members to tell them what was going on. During surgery, they removed any infected tissue, which included Bridget's left breast, and part of her back and side; they were able to save her left arm. She remained hospitalized for almost a month, and had several more months of recuperation at home.

Though Bridget survived, her physicians told her that her decision to go to the doctor that day saved her life. If the infection had spread a bit farther into her chest wall, they likely would not have been able to save her, as her heart would have been affected. As it was, she ended up with a 16-inch scar and numbness in her arm, but she was alive.

The term *invasive*, when applied to infectious diseases, has a very specific meaning. Most infections are termed localized, which means they occur in a specific area of the body (for example, in a cut on the hand). The infectious agent does not travel through the body to infect other areas. However, an **invasive disease** is unique in that the microbe has breached the body's basic defenses, and has spread throughout the body. The most common way for this to occur is for the microbe to gain access to the host's bloodstream; from there it can travel throughout the host's body, searching for a suitable place to reproduce and establish a new infection, often causing the host great harm along the way. The most common invasive infections caused by the group A streptococcus are bacteremia, streptococcal toxic shock syndrome, necrotizing fasciitis, and myositis.

BACTEREMIA

Bacteremia (presence of bacteria in the blood) is the most common of the invasive diseases caused by group A streptococcus bacteria. This can have a variety of symptoms and outcomes. Occasionally, no symptoms are seen. Most often, the patient will show fever and lethargy, similar to a bout of influenza. Though bacteremia is a disease on its own, it often can lead to other severe diseases (including those described later in this chapter) as the bacteria travel throughout the host's bloodstream and find new areas in which to reproduce.

Traditionally, streptococcal bacteremia has occurred in very young and very old people, most often in those with underlying conditions that may reduce the body's natural ability to resist disease. However, more recently, intravenous drug use has emerged as a leading cause of GABHS bacteremia in people between the ages of 14 and 40 (previously, the only significant cause of bacteremia in this age group was puerperal sepsis). In a study carried out in Norway, P. R. Martin and E. A. Hoiby demonstrated that the age group with the greatest increase in prevalence of GAS bacteremia in the late 1980s was adolescents and young adults—who showed an amazing 600–800% increase in the incidence of bacteremia during this decade. This correlates with the increase in other invasive diseases caused by the group A streptococcus that were observed during this same period. Currently, approximately 8,500 cases of GABHS bacteremia occur in the United States each year (approximately 3 cases per 100,000 people).

STREPTOCOCCAL TOXIC SHOCK SYNDROME

By the 1970s serious diseases caused by group A streptococci were thought to be all but vanquished in developed countries. Scarlet fever had essentially disappeared from the United States and many European countries. Many nations discontinued the practice of routinely administering antibiotics to army recruits, which had been used to prevent outbreaks of streptococcal disease.

However, by the mid-1980s epidemiologists and physicians noted a resurgence of severe diseases caused by *Streptococcus pyogenes*. Systemic diseases with severe complications were reported with increasing frequency. Outbreaks of rheumatic fever (a postinfectious sequelae of streptococcal infection) were also noted in different areas.

In the late 1970s a disease called **toxic shock syndrome** (**TSS**) first appeared. Although TSS has some clinical features similar to scarlet fever (fever, rash, peeling of the skin from the palms of the hands and the soles of the feet), it did

TOXIC SHOCK SYNDROME AND SUPERABSORBENT TAMPONS: PREQUEL TO INVASIVE STREPTOCOCCAL DISEASE

Early in American history, women used a variety of devices, including rags, cloth diaper-like contraptions, or home-rolled cotton sticks, to absorb menstrual fluid. However, when women began to enter the workforce, none of these methods seemed adequate. Therefore, when a Denver physician developed the first tampon in 1936, women eagerly turned to this alternative. By the 1960s tampons were in widespread use worldwide.

Tampons, however, were still not perfect, and women still had to deal with unpleasant leaks. Thus, tampon manufacturers worked to increase absorbency. In 1979 Procter & Gamble released a tampon that was capable of absorbing nearly 20 times its own weight in fluid. Other companies followed suit, releasing their own superabsorbent tampons.

The new tampons were actually able to absorb more fluid than most women had in their vaginas at a given time. Thus, the tampons effectively dried out the walls of the vagina and even adhered to the vaginal walls. In some cases the tampons tore cells from the vaginal wall when they were removed, causing pain and increasing the risk of infection. In extreme cases, medical intervention was necessary to remove the tampon.

In the early 1980s physicians noticed an increase in a disease known as toxic shock syndrome. About 95% of the cases were in females, and of those, almost all were menstruating women. The bacterium *Staphylococcus aureus* was cultured from most of the women. It was eventually determined that a new strain of *Staphylococcus aureus* had emerged, carrying a new, deadly toxin. The environment of the vagina and the superabsorbent tampons supplied an excellent area for these bacteria to multiply. Initially, women were warned to avoid using all tampons. Eventually, warning material was included in each box of tampons to educate women on how to use them safely. Fatalities from TSS decreased, just in time for a more lethal form of the disease, caused by the group A streptococcus, to break onto the scene.

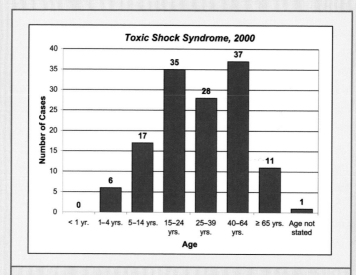

Figure 5.1 This graph shows the number of cases of toxic shock syndrome in the United States in the year 2000. Note that the highest rate of disease are among older teenagers and young adults (from age 15 to 24) and adults ages 40 to 64. (Centers for Disease Control and Prevention)

not affect the same group of patients that scarlet fever had. Rather, TSS almost exclusively affected women between the ages of 20 and 40, with a mortality rate of approximately 3%. This disease was eventually traced to a toxin-producing variant of the bacterium *Staphylococcus aureus*, a gram-positive coccus with many similarities to *Streptococcus pyogenes*. The disease was linked to the use of certain types of tampons. When the tampons were removed from the market, cases of TSS decreased quickly.

However, in the mid-1980s, just as cases of TSS caused by *Staphylococcus aureus* were decreasing, outbreaks of a disease with similar symptoms began to be reported. Patients were dying quickly of systemic shock, similar to the disease manifestation caused by *Staphylococcus aureus* and resulting in toxic shock syndrome. Logically, tampons were investigated initially as a **risk factor** for the disease. In these new outbreaks, however, patients did not have a history of tampon use. In fact, it was found that the infections causing these new outbreaks were not caused by *Staphylococcus aureus* at all; rather, they were found to be caused by group A streptococci. The disease was termed streptococcal toxic shock syndrome (STSS), to differentiate it from the similar disease caused by the *Staphylococcus aureus*. The appearance of a new disease caused by group A streptococci led the CDC to classify the group A streptococcus as a **reemerging pathogen.**

Fatality due to severe shock and organ failure could quickly ensue (within hours after the development of symptoms). Depending on the hospital, between 30 and 70% of patients with STSS died despite aggressive modern treatments. As with many diseases, if the patient was diagnosed and treated very quickly following the onset of symptoms, he or she was more likely to survive the disease, and the fatality rate varied depending on both the doctor and the hospital. What was unique about the profile of the patients diagnosed with STSS was that many were found to be otherwise healthy adults. In contrast, earlier cases of group A streptococcus (GAS) bacteremia most often occurred in patients who were under age 10 or older than 60, and most had underlying conditions, such as cancer or compromised immune systems, that made them more susceptible to disease. The fact that a new, fatal illness was striking the young and healthy was a cause for alarm in medical circles.

The way various patients acquired the strain of GAS associated with STSS, in many cases, remains a mystery. Most commonly, infection began at a site of a minor local injury, such as a cut, scrape, or bruise. In some cases it appears that the bacteria were able to gain access to the circulatory system because of damage by a preexisting virus, such as influenza or varicella (chicken pox). In general, cases of STSS have occurred sporadically, although a few large outbreaks have been reported.

The most common initial symptom of STSS is severe pain, which is often abrupt in onset. Fever is another frequent early sign. In approximately 10 percent of patients, a scarlet fever–like rash may be present. Blood pressure may also drop rapidly, leading to shock, organ failure, and death. Additionally, in 80 percent of STSS patients, clinical signs of soft tissue infection are present. This may progress to necrotizing fasciitis, a deep tissue infection that may lead to death.

"FLESH-EATING DISEASE": NECROTIZING FASCIITIS

Necrotizing fasciitis (NF) is a third invasive disease caused by the group A streptococcus. STSS and NF can be mutually exclusive (one can occur without the other), but in most patients, they appear together, and death results from organ system failure.

The condition known as necrotizing fasciitis (dubbed "the flesh-eating disease" by the media, and previously known as "streptococcal gangrene") is a serious disease characterized by a deep-seated infection of the **subcutaneous** tissue, which

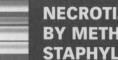

NECROTIZING FASCIITIS CAUSED BY METHICILLIN-RESISTANT STAPHYLOCOCCUS AUREUS (MRSA)

While GABHS remains the most common cause of necrotizing fasciitis, NF caused by another bacterium, *Staphylococcus aureus,* has increased over the past decade, mirroring an increase in the amount of MRSA present in the general population. In one hospital in Denver, Colorado, all patients with NF were examined from January 2004 to February 2006 to determine the microbial cause of their infection. Of 30 NF cases during this time period, five were caused by MRSA. Most patients reported a "spider bite" lesion 2–3 days prior to onset of NF, which is a common feature of community-associated MRSA infections. All MRSA strains were found to be the USA300 strain, which is the most common type of MRSA carried by individuals lacking hospital contact. ("Hospital-associated" strains of MRSA, such as USA100, are more common in medical centers such as hospitals and nursing homes, but these are rarely seen in individuals who have not been involved in health care.) As USA300 spreads through the population, we can expect to see more NF caused by this organism.[1]

progressively destroys fat and fascia, but often spares the skin and muscle. The initial signs of necrotizing fasciitis may include localized swelling (**edema**) and a feeling of warmth in the affected area (**erythema**). The patient may notice a cut, bruise, scratch, or boil in the tender area. The patient may also have a fever, sore throat, chills, and body aches. All of these symptoms are similar to those of influenza, and the patient often mistakes them for the flu and delays treatment as the infection worsens.

A day or two after the onset of symptoms, the pain in the affected area may progress from being an occasional annoyance to unbearable agony. The area may appear bright red and shiny to the touch. As more time passes, the area will become purple or almost black in color. If the infection is found at this point,

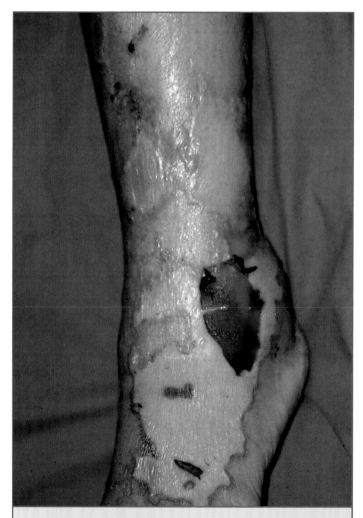

Figure 5.2 Necrotizing fasciitis, shown here on the leg and foot, causes rapid degeneration of the skin and fascia. This disease can spread through the tissue at the rate of an inch an hour. Often the only treatment is to amputate the affected body part. (© Dr. Ken Greer/Visuals Unlimited, Inc./Getty Images)

generally, surgical removal of the whole affected area will be required. In extreme cases an entire limb may need to be amputated to halt the spread of infection, which can be quite rapid; the progression of infection at the rate of an inch an hour has been documented. If not yet diagnosed or treated, by this point, the patient's blood pressure often will have dropped. The heart rate will increase in an attempt to pump more blood to the organs (this rapid heartbeat is termed **tachycardia**). The final symptoms of NF are similar to STSS, as the body's organs shut down due to a lack of blood supply. Without treatment, death from NF is certain.

STREPTOCOCCAL MYOSITIS

Streptococcal myositis is an extremely rare disease. In fact, there have been only 25 documented cases worldwide between the years of 1950 and 2000. However, the fatality rate attributed to the disease is exceedingly high; depending on the speed and effectiveness of treatment, between 80 and 100% of patients eventually succumb to the disease.[2] Streptococcal myositis is different from necrotizing fasciitis in that the bacteria that cause the infection invade and destroy the muscle; they do not stop at the skin and fascia. This makes the infection much more invasive—and much more deadly. Again, streptococcal myositis may be the result of a complication of streptococcal toxic shock-like syndrome, and may also be present with necrotizing fasciitis (in which case, the bacteria would invade and destroy the fascia, the fat, and the muscle). Myositis may also be caused by bacteremia, even if the patient suffered only mild symptoms during the initial infection. The only cure for streptococcal myositis is surgery to remove the damaged tissue entirely in order to prevent the infection from spreading further.

6

Post-Streptococcal Complications

After three weeks, Bongani was finally recovering from his illness—a flu-like infection that had left him largely unable to help his family for the better part of a week. Bongani, the oldest of six children, hated not being able to help his father—he liked being depended on, and felt proud that he was a very responsible son. He had hoped to feel fully recovered by today, but just when his throat was feeling better and he was regaining his energy, he woke up to find his left knee stiff and painful and slightly red in color. His mother, who had come to see why he wasn't out of bed yet, grimaced when he described his symptoms. She recognized them, as rheumatic fever is common in their village. Though she only knew the local name rather than the scientific one, Bongani's illness had likely been caused by GABHS, and the joint stiffness and swelling in his knee were the first symptoms of rheumatic fever. She called for Bongani's father, and together they started the long walk toward the nearest clinic, almost three hours away by foot. There, Bongani would receive antibiotics, but the doctor would warn his father that it may be too late—that the damage may already be irreversible and unable to be stopped at this point. The doctor told them to closely monitor any other symptoms Bongani develops, as rheumatic fever can lead to rheumatic heart disease, one of the most common causes of cardiac disease in Africa. Damage to Bongani's heart could leave him weak and unable to carry out necessary tasks as he ages; the worst-case scenario, Bongani's doctor tells his father, is death.

In many situations, the invading group A streptococci are treated with antibiotics and killed, ending the bacteria's effects on the person who was infected. However, the effects on the human host do not always stop when the invading bacteria are killed and the infection is cleared. Indeed, for some people, the worst effects of these bacteria appear after the infection has cleared the body. The inclusive term for these effects of the bacterial infection is *postinfection sequelae*, meaning that the conditions occur after the active infection has ceased. Although the bacteria may no longer be present in the patient's body, the effects of the brief infection can be long-lasting and even deadly.

RHEUMATIC FEVER AND RHEUMATIC HEART DISEASE

One such post-infection sequel is rheumatic fever, a disease that affects multiple organs and systems, including the heart, joints, central nervous system, subcutaneous tissue, and skin. This disease most frequently strikes children between the ages of 5 and 15. Generally, the first clinical signs of rheumatic fever are fever and arthritis in the joints.

Rheumatic fever can damage the heart valves, causing them to fail to close properly or not open wide enough. When a valve fails to close properly, it allows blood to leak backward. When a valve does not open wide enough, the heart must pump harder to force blood through the narrowed opening. When damage to the heart is permanent, the condition is called **rheumatic heart disease** (or **rheumatic carditis**), a common consequence of rheumatic fever. Rheumatic heart disease occurs in about half of rheumatic fever patients, generally within three weeks of the onset of symptoms.

Cases of rheumatic fever and rheumatic heart disease occur most often in developing countries. Estimates suggest that between 10 and 20 million new cases of rheumatic fever occur each year in such areas. In addition, rheumatic heart disease is the leading cause of death from cardiac disease among individuals younger than age 40 in developing countries. In Brazil alone, between 8,000 and 10,000 cardiac surgeries are performed each year to treat rheumatic heart disease and similar rheumatic fever sequelae.

Some rheumatic fever patients may show neurological symptoms, called **Sydenham chorea**. All such diseases are thought to result from an interaction of certain strains of GABHS and a particular **genotype** (genetic makeup) of the host.

DISCOVERING THE CAUSE OF RHEUMATIC FEVER

Investigation into the **etiology** of rheumatic fever began more than a century ago. Two German scientists, Hugo Schottmuller and Béla Schick, made significant contributions to the initial investigation in the early part of the twentieth century. Schottmuller differentiated between hemolytic and nonhemolytic groups of streptococci by growing bacteria on blood agar plates. Schick, meanwhile, recognized by 1912 that both rheumatic fever and acute glomerulonephritis occurred after infection with scarlet fever. However, it would take another 25 years after Schick's studies to confirm that, indeed, group A streptococci were the cause of scarlet fever, partly due to work carried out by Alvin Coburn in the early 1930s.

By the early 1930s studies had suggested that rheumatic fever was a sequel to GAS pharyngitis and rarely to other GAS superficial diseases, such as impetigo. In addition, investigators discovered that not all strains of GABHS were capable of causing rheumatic fever, even if they were isolated from a throat infection. This discovery led to the realization that some strains were **rheumatagenic** (capable of causing rheumatic fever), while others were not. This difference was found to relate to the production of a protein called opacity factor, which, in turn, correlated to a certain class of M protein. In addition, scientists found that environmental and host factors played a role in the development of the disease.

By the late 1930s **sulfonamides** were shown to be effective in preventing recurrences of rheumatic fever. By the following decade, penicillin had come into widespread use. In a study carried out by Charles Rammelkamp and others, penicillin was shown to be effective at treating streptococcal pharyngitis and efficiently preventing initial attacks of rheumatic fever. Prescribing penicillin was considered such an effective preventive strategy that penicillin came to be administered prophylactically (as a precautionary measure) to all healthy army recruits, which essentially put an end to epidemics of streptococcal pharyngitis and rheumatic fever on military bases. This strategy was soon extended to the general population. Administering penicillin to anyone suspected of having streptococcal pharyngitis quickly reduced cases of rheumatic fever in the United States. High-quality health care and clean environments also served to decrease the incidence of rheumatic fever in developed countries. In fact, by the early 1980s, rheumatic fever had all but disappeared in the United States, Western Europe, Japan, and Australia, even though rates of streptococcal pharyngitis remained unchanged.

RESURGENCE OF RHEUMATIC FEVER

Because the incidence of rheumatic fever in the United States had been steadily dropping for almost half a century, many people were surprised when rheumatic fever made a sudden resurgence in the 1980s. One outbreak occurred at the San Diego Naval Base; another at Fort Leonard Wood, Missouri; and yet another among schoolchildren in several other regions of the United States. Unlike the rheumatic fever outbreaks of a century before, these epidemics were not related to overcrowding, poverty, or uncleanliness (indeed, most occurred in middle- or upper-class neighborhoods). Two serotypes (classification of strains of group A streptococci based on the M protein)—M18 and M3—were prominent in these outbreaks. In addition, bacteria isolated from these populations were found to produce large amounts of **capsule**, an extracellular coating produced by some isolates of GAS. These heavily encapsulated, mucoid strains had not been seen for decades, but were previously associated with military rheumatic fever epidemics.

Finally, although the incidence of rheumatic fever and its associated complications in the United States has increased in recent decades, deaths from these diseases are still relatively rare. In 2000 approximately 3,500 deaths were caused by rheumatic fever and rheumatic heart disease (fewer than 1.5 cases per 100,000 people). In contrast, there were 15,000 such deaths in 1950.

The presence of virulent strains of GABHS in the population has played a role in the rise and fall of rheumatic fever outbreaks, but factors relating to the host and environment also play a role in the development of this, and other, streptococcal postinfection sequelae.

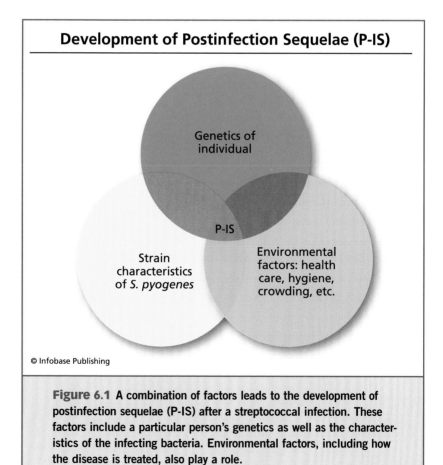

Development of Postinfection Sequelae (P-IS)

Genetics of individual

P-IS

Strain characteristics of *S. pyogenes*

Environmental factors: health care, hygiene, crowding, etc.

© Infobase Publishing

Figure 6.1 A combination of factors leads to the development of postinfection sequelae (P-IS) after a streptococcal infection. These factors include a particular person's genetics as well as the characteristics of the infecting bacteria. Environmental factors, including how the disease is treated, also play a role.

HOST FACTORS AND RHEUMATIC FEVER

Some properties of bacteria have been suggested to play a role in the development of rheumatic fever, but host factors also may be a key factor in determining whether a person recovering from a streptococcal infection will suffer this postinfection sequel. Both rheumatic fever and acute post-streptococcal glomerulonephritis are considered **autoimmune diseases**; this means they are diseases that result from the body's immune system attacking the body's own cells rather than attacking invading microbes. It is unclear exactly what triggers this aberrant response or why it develops in some patients but not in others. The hypothesis that individual host factors are involved in the development of these diseases was strengthened with the discovery of the **major histocompatibility complex (MHC)** class of proteins. These proteins are a part of the human immune system and are involved in the recognition of foreign proteins, such as those on the surface of bacterial cells. In some studies, rheumatic fever has been shown to develop more frequently in individuals who have a certain MHC type; presently, it is not known exactly why these individuals develop the disease more often. In addition, studies linking particular MHC types to rheumatic fever have been contradictory, and the results remain inconclusive. Further studies into this matter are currently being conducted.

BACTERIAL FACTORS AND RHEUMATIC FEVER

The third important factor in the development of rheumatic fever is the properties of the infecting bacteria themselves. As outlined above, certain serotypes of GABHS are more likely to cause rheumatic fever or rheumatic heart disease than other serotypes are. In the United States, the most common serotypes that have been documented to cause rheumatic fever are types 1, 3, 5, 6, 18, 19, and 24. It has been hypothesized that the protein responsible for specifying the serotype, the **M protein**, plays a particularly important role in rheumatic heart disease. This protein has a coiled structure similar to cardiac **myosin**, a protein present in the heart. Therefore, it is possible that antibodies that are formed against the

M protein during an infection may also (erroneously) bind to cardiac myosin, triggering an immune response against this critical host protein (called an **antigenic cross-reaction**). Again, the results of studies to test this hypothesis have been inconclusive.

ACUTE POST-STREPTOCOCCAL GLOMERULONEPHRITIS

The term *glomerulonephritis* describes a group of diseases characterized by inflammatory changes in glomerular capillaries (small blood vessels in the **glomeruli**, the filtering tubules that make up the kidneys). It has a number of causes. When an antecedent streptococcal infection causes glomerulonephritis, the disease is called **acute post-streptococcal glomerulonephritis (APSGN)**. This disease occurs approximately 14–21 days after infection with a **nephritogenic** strain of GABHS ("nephritogenic" strains have been identified in a similar manner to "rheumatogenic" strains.

Although many studies have been done on APSGN, scientists at the present time know little about the way the disease begins. It is known that the disease often follows a respiratory tract infection with GABHS if the patient lives in a cold climate, and typically follows a group A streptococcal skin infection if the patient lives in a warmer climate. The reason for the difference in initial infections is not known.

Although invasive diseases caused by the group A streptococcus, as well as the incidence of rheumatic fever, have increased during the past decade in developed countries, a similar increase in cases of APSGN has not been observed. However, in other areas of the world, APSGN is common, particularly in places with tropical climates where streptococcal skin infections often occur. For example, in Africa and Hong Kong, streptococcal infection is almost the only cause of acute glomerulonephritis in children.

HOST FACTORS AND APSGN

Little is currently known about the role of host factors in the development of APSGN. However, epidemiological studies have shown that the disease most often appears in individuals with certain socioeconomic backgrounds and people of a certain age and gender. Therefore, some factors that make individuals more susceptible to the disease are likely to be involved. As with rheumatic fever, a person's MHC type has been linked to the development of disease; however, the studies are inconclusive at this time.

ENVIRONMENTAL FACTORS AND APSGN

It has also been determined that outbreaks of the disease occur in crowded areas where poor hygiene, malnutrition, and parasitic infections are commonplace. For example, an epidemic of APSGN involving 474 patients occurred in Armenia between 1992 and 1996. This epidemic happened after an abrupt economic decline in the country, which began in 1990 and led to poor living conditions, including a lack of heated homes and absence of routine medical care. Poor hygiene led to an increase in streptococcal skin infections and the postinfection sequelae that may follow.

BACTERIAL FACTORS AND ASPGN

Numerous bacterial factors have been implicated as potentially being involved in the development of APSGN. Again, the most commonly cited factor is the M protein. Serotypes most often associated with APSGN include M types 1, 4, 12, 49, 55, 57, and 60. However, not all isolates of these serotypes are associated with APSGN; rather, it appears to be a strain-specific property. Also, some experts believe certain portions of these M proteins are similar in structure to proteins present in the glomeruli. Just as with the case of M proteins and cardiac myosin, the structural similarity between the M proteins and glomeruli may result in an antigenic cross-reaction in which antibodies that are supposed to target the invading bacteria's M proteins target instead the host's own proteins, causing severe damage.

It has also been hypothesized that APSGN is caused by the deposition of **antigen-antibody complexes** (associations between

Kidney and Nephron

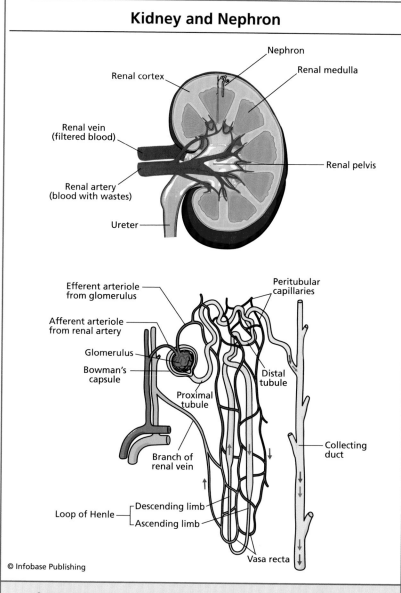

Nephron
Renal cortex
Renal medulla
Renal vein (filtered blood)
Renal pelvis
Renal artery (blood with wastes)
Ureter

Efferent arteriole from glomerulus
Peritubular capillaries
Afferent arteriole from renal artery
Glomerulus
Bowman's capsule
Distal tubule
Proximal tubule
Branch of renal vein
Collecting duct
Loop of Henle — Descending limb / Ascending limb
Vasa recta

© Infobase Publishing

Figure 6.2 Above is a diagram of a kidney in cross-section, and below is a close-up view of a nephron. Scientists believe that glomerulonephritis may result after antigen-antibody complexes are deposited in the individual glomeruli of the kidneys.

portions of the bacterial proteins—antigens—and the host's defense molecules—antibodies) in the glomeruli, which, in turn, may lead to inflammation and tissue damage. Studies have shown that these deposits may happen late in the disease process, but that this is likely not the initial cause.

NEUROPSYCHIATRIC DISORDERS

The role GABHS plays in the etiology of diseases such as rheumatic fever and glomerulonephritis has been well established, if not well understood. Interestingly, recent lines of investigation have suggested that GABHS may play a role in far more diseases than we are currently aware. In the past decade, there has been an increasing recognition by many investigators that microbial infections are involved in the development of a wide range of chronic diseases, ranging from peptic ulcer disease to cancer. Some researchers believe that several neuropsychiatric disorders of childhood may also be rooted in a microbe-triggered autoimmune response, similar to that seen in the development of the diseases described above.

A potential connection has been found between infection with GABHS and neuropsychiatric disorders, such as Tourette syndrome, obsessive-compulsive disorder, and possibly attention-deficit/hyperactivity disorder (ADHD). Patients with these conditions have some biological markers that are similar to those observed in rheumatic fever patients. Furthermore, one manifestation of rheumatic fever, known as Sydenham chorea, is characterized by symptoms similar to those observed in patients with Tourette syndrome. Sydenham chorea is a nonprogressive neurological movement disorder that includes spontaneous movements, lack of coordination of voluntary movements, and muscular weakness. Interestingly, this disease targets the basal ganglia of the brain, which is also the area targeted in Tourette syndrome, obsessive-compulsive disorder, and attention-deficit/hyperactivity disorder. This evidence suggests that the diseases may have a common cause: infection with the group A streptococcus. Since the role that

SYDENHAM, THE "ENGLISH HIPPOCRATES"

Thomas Sydenham (1624–1689), an English-born physician, has been dubbed the "English Hippocrates." He believed it was the state of the atmosphere and the hypothetical changes within it that produced disease, a phenomenon he called "the epidemic constitution." Sydenham believed that epidemics increased in severity as the epidemic constitution developed its force to the fullest; the epidemic would then decline as the atmospheric conditions changed to favor a new constitution. Although he was not clear on what he meant in terms of the atmospheric change, he thought the change was caused by a miasma arising from the earth. He even believed it was possible that epidemics had an astrological orgin.

These ideas may sound fanciful today, but the method by which Sydenham arrived at his conclusions was his greatest contribution to medicine. He made direct observations and painstakingly described symptoms and environmental conditions to differentiate between diseases that had similar clinical presentations. He was one of the first physicians to use cinchona bark (which contains quinine, the basis for modern-day antimalarial drugs) to treat malaria. He described conditions including gout, smallpox, malaria, scarlet fever, and Sydenham chorea (which now bears his name) in great detail. Sydenham established himself as the father of modern clinical medicine and epidemiology.

GABHS plays in Sydenham chorea has been known for many years, researchers have hypothesized that perhaps these bacteria are also involved in the development of Tourette syndrome. The association between GABHS infection and these neuropsychiatric disorders, called pediatric autoimmune neuropsychiatric disorders associated with streptococcal infections (**PANDAS**), is an area of active investigation.

Initial studies of PANDAS have provided some interesting results. Approximately 70% of patients with Sydenham chorea have reported that they experienced an onset of repetitive, unwanted thoughts and behaviors before their chorea began, similar to the experience of patients with childhood-onset obsessive-compulsive disorder. This suggests that Sydenham chorea and obsessive-compulsive disorder may have a common cause: GABHS. Other studies have found significantly increased rates of rheumatic fever among the parents or grandparents of children who have been diagnosed with either Sydenham chorea or PANDAS. Thus, these data suggest that children in the PANDAS group may have inherited a susceptibility to post-streptococcal sequelae similar to that reported for children with Sydenham chorea. Other studies have shown that children who have been diagnosed with PANDAS have increased rates of obsessive-compulsive disorder and **tics** among their family members. This, too, suggests a dual role of infection by GABHS as well as genetic makeup as being necessary to develop the disease symptoms. Proof of this connection awaits additional testing and research.

7

Virulence Factors of Group A Streptococci

Bacteria have been a threat to human health for as long as we have been around. Therefore, the body has developed many different mechanisms to protect itself from infection by bacteria.

GENERAL PHYSICAL AND CHEMICAL DEFENSES TO INFECTION

Our bodies have a number of physical barriers that impede bacterial infection. These serve as the "first line" of defense. The first and most obvious is our epithelium: our outer covering or skin, as well as the epithelial cells that line our mouth, nose, respiratory, digestive, urinary, and reproductive tracts. This defense works in two ways. First, it is a simple barrier. Second, it is constantly regenerated: Any bacteria that are attached to the dead cells are sloughed off as these old cells are replaced by new cells. However, any time we have a cut or scratch, that barrier is breached, and may serve as a portal for bacteria to enter other areas of our body through our bloodstream. Our epithelium is already covered with microbes. These bacteria generally do not make us sick; they are termed **normal flora** (meaning that it is normal for them to be there). They serve an important purpose by simply taking up space—space that otherwise could be occupied by more dangerous species of bacteria.

Another physical defense is the presence of **mucus**. Most of the exposed areas of our respiratory and digestive tracts are covered in mucus. This serves as a type of "trap" for bacteria. They become stuck in the mucus layer, and are unable to gain access to our body tissue. Additionally, there are **antibodies** (special proteins produced by the human **immune system** to combat pathogens) and chemicals as well as cells within in the mucus which are able to kill bacteria. These cells are termed **phagocytes**.

Other physical defenses include the presence of **ciliated cells** in the airways in our lungs (ciliated cells have a tail-like instrument and act together to move bacteria up the respiratory tract in order to remove them from the lungs), the presence of acid in the stomach (which will kill many bacteria, if they are swallowed), and the presence of antimicrobial chemicals in tears. Movement (of air, as in the lungs; or of fluid or solids, as in the mouth, urinary tract, and intestine) also serves to prevent bacteria from attaching to cells of the body and beginning an infection.

IMMUNE DEFENSES

Though our physical defenses work to keep us healthy most of the time, bacteria are occasionally able to get by. When this happens, the body's immune system takes over. An early immune response increases the number of phagocytes in the vicinity of the invading bacteria. *Phagocyte* is a generic term for a group of cells that kill bacteria by engulfing and "eating" them.

More specific immune defenses important to group A streptococcal infection include **complement** and antibodies. Complement is the name given to a group of proteins that are present in the blood. Complement can either act on its own, assembling on the surface of the bacterium and creating a structure that literally pokes holes in the bacterium and leads to its death, or can do the same thing more quickly and efficiently in conjunction with antibodies.

Antibodies are another type of protein present in the blood, which are produced by special cells, called **B cells**. Antibodies are very specific, and each one recognizes a different portion of proteins produced by specific bacteria. This specific portion

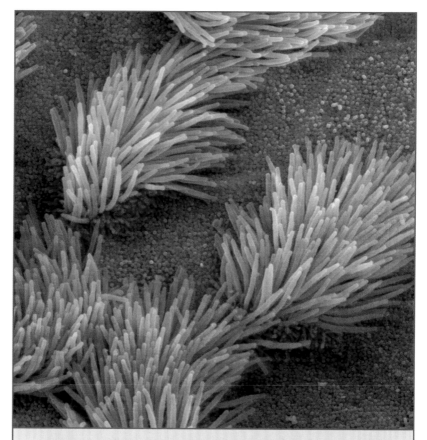

Figure 7.1 This electron micrograph shows the cilia on lung cells. These projections serve to trap microbes and move them up and out of the lung. By removing foreign particles, the cilia act as an important barrier to infection. (© RMF/Visuals Unlimited, Inc./Getty Images)

is termed the **antigen**. It takes several days for the body to produce these specific antibodies when a new pathogen is encountered, so these are more important late in the infection. When antibody molecules find a foreign protein (an antigen) they recognize, they bind to it. This then signals phagocytic cells to engulf and destroy the bacterium. Although phagocytes can do this on their own, they do it much more efficiently when the bacteria are coated with antibody.

Many bacteria have evolved efficient mechanisms in order to escape these various host defenses. In **pathogenic** bacteria (bacteria that cause disease), the factors that allow the organism to avoid the host's various defenses are often termed **virulence factors**.

WHAT IS VIRULENCE?

The virulence of a pathogen refers to the severity of the clinical illness that results from infection. Since the symptoms caused by the infection (such as fever, swelling, and pain) are actually a by-product of the immune response, pathogens that fail to provoke an immune response will cause no clinical signs of disease. For example, the bacteria mentioned above as "normal flora" are rarely virulent: Under normal circumstances, they provoke no immune response from the host, and do not breach any of the host's first-line defenses. Virulence factors, therefore, are any features of bacteria that allow them to cause a clinical infection.

The overall virulence of populations of bacteria also may change over years or decades. For example, during the mid-twentieth century, group A streptococci appeared to be evolving into less harmful bacteria. What had been a major cause of morbidity and mortality in the early part of the century had become an easily treatable infection that was rarely a serious concern. However, the epidemiology of GABHS infections rapidly changed beginning in the mid-1980s. Today, these bacteria cause a variety of severe illnesses.

In addition, virulence is not dependent on bacterial factors alone. Several host factors have been shown to increase the risk of severe invasive streptococcal disease. A person's age, whether the person has any underlying disease, and whether the person has an ongoing viral infection can determine the likelihood that the person will develop severe disease when infected with GAS. Even in a healthy human, the person's immune responses to different streptococcal virulence factors can vary. Lack of **protective immunity** (previous exposure to the pathogen, which allows for a quicker antibody response when the same pathogen enters the

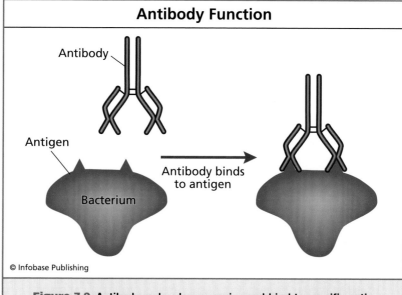

Antibody Function

Antibody

Antigen

Bacterium

Antibody binds
to antigen

© Infobase Publishing

Figure 7.2 Antibody molecules recognize and bind to specific antigens on bacterial cells. Then, other immune cells (such as phagocytes) target and kill the antibody-coated bacterium, which helps eliminate the infection.

body, protecting the host from reinfection) to specific virulence factors produced by bacteria is likely to affect host susceptibility to infection. Studies have suggested that these varied responses may help explain why some people develop severe disease and others only mild cases, even if they are infected with the same strain of GABHS.

SPECIFIC VIRULENCE FACTORS
IN GROUP A STREPTOCOCCI

One of the most important virulence factors to be discovered in the group A streptococcus is the **M protein**. M proteins are multifunctional proteins on the cell surface that play a role in bacterial resistance to **phagocytosis**, increase adherence to host tissues (that is, allow the bacteria to "stick" to host cells), and also make it easier for the bacteria to invade host cells (this is a way the bacteria may "hide" from the host's immune system—by entering the host's own cells). Because of the various roles these proteins play, possibly at different stages during the infection, they have been deemed a critical virulence factor of GABHS.

Rebecca Lancefield first described the M protein of GAS in 1928. This protein extends from the cell surface and appears as fibrils (thin, fiber-like structures) on the surface of group A streptococci. Antibodies to M proteins identified different serotypes of these bacteria. Lancefield's studies formed the basis for attributing an **antiphagocytic** role to the M protein (meaning that it prevents the uptake and killing of the bacteria by phagocytes) and established the M protein as a major virulence factor of GAS. Lancefield determined this by carrying out experiments in which the only difference between two populations of bacteria was the presence of M protein on the surface. She found that those bacteria that lacked M protein were quickly phagocytosed (taken up and eliminated by phagocytic cells) and destroyed, while those that produced M protein were less likely to be killed by the host, and were more likely to establish a clinical infection and cause harm to the host.

Recently, analysis of the genes coding for the M proteins (termed *emm* genes) has shown that these are members of a larger *emm*-like gene family. This means that there are genes similar in sequence to the *emm* gene close by on the bacterial chromosome. A gene that encodes a protein called **C5a peptidase** (a protein that cuts up and destroys a complement protein; it is encoded by a gene named *scpA*) is also present in this region of the chromosome, which is termed the **Mga regulon**. (A regulon is a group of several genes that are all subject to a common regulator—that is, a gene that controls the production of the proteins encoded by the rest of the genes in the regulon.) All the genes in this region encode proteins that interfere with functions of the host's immune system; therefore, they have been ascribed a role in enhancing the virulence of GABHS.

Opacity Factor Isolates of *Streptococcus pyogenes*

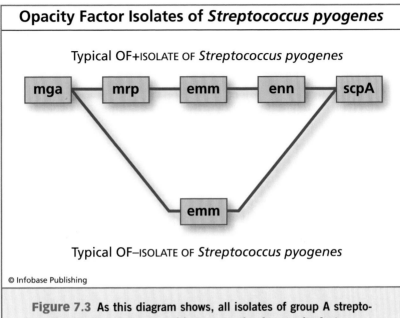

Typical OF+ISOLATE OF *Streptococcus pyogenes*

Typical OF–ISOLATE OF *Streptococcus pyogenes*

© Infobase Publishing

Figure 7.3 As this diagram shows, all isolates of group A streptococci—whether they are positive or negative for opacity factor— have a regulon that begins with the mga gene and ends with the *scpA* gene.

THE M PROTEINS AND *EMM* GENES

Strains of GABHS can be distinguished from each other by using a serotyping method to determine which type of M protein each bacterium expresses. The reason this works is because, as a population, GABHS possess many different *emm* **alleles** (forms of the same gene). This means that, as a group, they will express M proteins (encoded by the *emm* genes) that vary slightly in their structure. Most of this variability is found at the tip of the protein that is farthest from the cell surface. Since this is where the antibodies contact the cell, it is to the advantage of the bacterial population to have a good deal of variability present in the **amino acid** sequence (the building blocks of proteins) of different M proteins expressed by different strains of GABHS. For example, if the host has already encountered a **strain** of GABHS of the same serotype in the past—for example, serotype 1—the host will already have antibodies against that serotype of bacterium. It will be difficult or impossible for any bacteria that carry a serotype 1 M protein to establish an infection in that host. The host is said to be **immune** to that particular serotype of bacteria. However, a bacterium carrying an M protein of a different serotype (for example, serotype 18) will not be recognized by the host, and may consequently cause an infection. Therefore, it is an advantage to the population of GABHS to maintain a lot of diversity in regard to M protein sequence. This increases the chances of being able to establish a successful infection in the host.

Although there is a large amount of diversity in the M protein sequence in GABHS, investigators have separated all these different types of M proteins into two general classes: class I and class II M proteins. Class II M proteins are typically associated with the presence of another Mga-regulated gene, called

REGULATION OF GENES BY MGA

Research during the past decade has identified a positive regulator of the M protein expression in group A streptococci. This means that a gene was discovered (the *mga* gene) whose product, the Mga protein, increases the creation of the protein products of other genes in the Mga regulon. Therefore, when the Mga protein is produced, it increases the amount of proteins made by the *emm*, *mrp*, *enn*, *scpA*, and *sic* genes. Scientists have also done experiments to show that there is a negative regulator of these genes, too. This negative regulator acts as an "off" switch, decreasing expression of these genes, while the positive regulator is like a switch set to the "on" position. One such negative regulator gene has been identified, called *covS*.

Why are these regulatory genes necessary? Some experts think variety in surface structures (such as the M protein) is important for allowing pathogens to adapt to changing host *sof* (encoding the enzyme serum **opacity factor,** a protein that, when present, causes serum—the clear portion of blood—to become cloudy). Strains of GABHS that have class II M proteins and the *sof* gene are referred to as being opacity-factor-positive (OF+). Strains of bacteria with class I M proteins generally lack opacity factor, and are termed opacity-factor-negative (OF-). Class II M proteins are also associated with the presence of *mrp* and *enn* genes (these encode the M-like proteins termed Mrp and Enn, respectively) in the Mga regulon. OF- strains have a greater variability in genes that may be found in the Mga regulon, but generally consist of only *mga,* an *emm* gene that encodes a class I M protein, and *scpA* (the gene that encodes the C5a peptidase). This distinction between M protein classes has clinical relevance as well: For example, patients who develop rheumatic fever almost always have been previously infected

environments. For example, the kind of surface structures needed to colonize the host at first may not be required or may even be cumbersome to the bacteria during later stages of infection. Surface molecules that keep the bacteria at a specific site in the host have to be altered if the organism wants to change location or move to a new host. Invasive pathogens often need one set of genes to gain access to the host and another set to spread and get past host defenses in the tissues or systemic circulation. Certain key virulence factors may actually be harmful for the organism, if they make the organism a targeted antigen when the host mounts an immune response. Therefore, once infection is established, the bacteria may express fewer virulence factors to avoid being killed off by the host. The regulatory genes are the keys to a quick switch for expressing or not expressing these virulence factors.[1]

with a strain of GABHS that carries a class I M protein, whereas more impetigo infections are caused by class II M proteins than by class I M proteins.

The M protein appears to play a role in the basic survival of GABHS. In the past, the group A streptococcus has tradition-ally been regarded as an **extracellular pathogen**. This means that, although it lives inside the host's body, it does not enter the individual cells of the host (with the exception of engulf-ment by phagocytic cells to destroy the bacteria). Rather, it lives either in the blood or on top of the host's cells. However, recent reports indicate that GABHS can promote its own uptake by a variety of mammalian cells, at least *in vitro* (outside of a living host). This means it may spend part of its time inside the host as an **intracellular pathogen** (living inside the host's cells). Evi-dence has accumulated to suggest that the ability to reside in an intracellular state can promote survival and dissemination of the bacterium within human populations. For example, beta-lactam antibiotics (such as penicillin), which do not readily enter the cells of mammals, fail to kill GABHS in up to 30% of children who have pharyngitis. Also, intracellular streptococci have been observed in tonsil cells under microscopic examina-tion, isolated from patients with recurrent pharyngitis. Several types of M proteins (1, 3, 6, and 18) have been found to pro-mote uptake of streptococci by host cells. Thus, entering the host's cells, a process facilitated by the M protein, appears to be an important survival strategy for some strains of GABHS.

THE "M-RELATED PROTEIN" (Mrp)

In addition to M proteins, there are a series of structurally related M-like proteins that form the *emm* **gene superfamily**. A given strain of group A streptococci may have one, two, or three *emm* or *emm*-like genes arranged in tandem on the chromosome near the positive transcriptional regulator, *mga*. These *emm* or *emm*-like genes encode for the M and M-like proteins, respectively. These M-like proteins have structural characteristics similar to those defined above for the M protein.

Genetic studies have suggested that a common ancestral gene has undergone gene duplication and divergence to produce the diversified family of M and M-like proteins.

Mrp is one M-like protein that is encoded by the *mrp* gene. This gene is located on the chromosome between the *emm* and *mga* genes. As with the M protein, the portion of the Mrp protein distal to the bacterial surface can vary between strains. Surface-expressed Mrp is thought to act much as the M protein does, by conferring antiphagocytic properties to streptococci growing in human blood. Though it appears to have the same function as M protein, it may be an advantage to the bacterium to be able to express these two different proteins (the M protein and the Mrp protein) at different stages of infection, in order to avoid attack by the host's antibodies. Both the M and Mrp proteins are believed to be most important for avoiding host defenses when infections occur on the skin or in the blood.

THE ENN PROTEIN

The *enn* gene, when present, is found between the *emm* and *scpA* genes on the chromosome, and encodes the M-like Enn protein. Like *mrp*, *enn* is associated with strains that are opacity-factor-positive. Unlike the Mrp and M proteins, Enn does not seem to have significant antiphagocytic properties. Rather, some researchers believe the Enn protein may help the bacteria resist the host's immune system during infections that occur on the **mucous membranes** rather than in the blood, as the M and Mrp proteins appear to do.

STREPTOCOCCAL C5a PEPTIDASE—*ScpA*

The final gene in the Mga regulon of both opacity factor positive and negative isolates is the *scpA* gene, which encodes a streptococcal C5a peptidase. This protein is a **protease** (a protein that cleaves and destroys other proteins; in this case, it destroys a host protein called C5a) present on the surface of the bacteria that is able to interfere with portions of the host's immune response.

Several lines of evidence suggest that the C5a peptidase plays an important role in the virulence of the group A streptococcus. First, all serotypes of GABHS tested to date produce a C5a peptidase or carry the *scpA* gene. Second, in laboratory experiments, mutations engineered in the *scpA* gene (which made the gene nonfunctional, and therefore unable to produce the C5a peptidase protein) increased the rate at which bacteria were killed in mice with **intranasal** (via the nose) infections. Third, when mice were given an intranasal vaccine made up of purified C5a peptidase protein, the mice were protected from further infection with GABHS. Finally, although fewer than 15% of children under 10 years of age exhibit measurable antibody against C5a peptidase, most adults have evidence of a strong immune response to the protein. This suggests that the host responds to this bacterial protein, and this response appears to protect the host from further infection with the group A streptococcus.

STREPTOCOCCAL INHIBITOR OF COMPLEMENT—*Sic*

Another gene that can be found in the Mga regulon of some OF- isolates encodes what is called the streptococcal inhibitor of complement-mediated lysis (Sic). This protein interferes with the complement proteins, preventing them from creating a hole in the bacterial membrane. When this gene is present in an isolate, it is generally found between the *emm* and *scpA* genes. Unlike most genes present in this region, the *sic* gene does not encode a surface protein (which the M, Mrp, and Enn proteins are). Rather, Sic is a secreted protein, meaning it is released from the cell.

Extensive screening of GABHS isolates has found that Sic was only present in a limited number of GABHS serotypes. In fact, thus far, only isolates of serotypes M1 and M57 have been found to contain the *sic* gene in their Mga regulon. Because many of the GAS isolates recovered from invasive disease in the previous decade have been of the M1 serotype, these data indicate that Sic could be an important virulence determinant. Additionally, many humans have been found to have antibodies in their blood that react specifically with portions of the Sic protein. Finally, experiments were done in which one group of mice was infected with *sic* mutants (the bacteria were unable to produce the Sic protein), while a second group of mice was infected with bacteria that produced Sic normally. It was found that the bacteria that were "normal" survived for a much longer period of time within the mice, whereas the bacteria that were unable to produce Sic were killed more quickly. This is likely to be important to the bacterium: If the bacteria are killed by the host's immune response too quickly after entering the host, they will be unable to start an infection and replicate within the host.

It should be noted that although investigators have discovered some functions that the proteins listed above may have during an infection of the host, others remain under investigation. The role these proteins play either alone or in combination with other bacterial products is actively being studied in a number of animal infection models.

OTHER VIRULENCE FACTORS: SUPERANTIGENS SpeA, SpeB, AND SpeC

Superantigens are proteins, produced by GABHS, that are able to alter the normal human immune response. This alteration leads to the increased production of host proteins called **cytokines**. These are chemicals that eventually may lead to the shock and multiorgan failure characteristic of streptococcal toxic shock syndrome (STSS). In the United States, STSS is frequently associated with strains of GABHS that produce the superantigen SpeA. These superantigens are also involved in the development of scarlet fever, and are responsible for the characteristic red rash and "strawberry tongue" symptomatic of that disease.

SpeA and SpeC are similar because the genes for these proteins are both encoded on **bacteriophages**—that is, on viruses that have become part of the streptococcus's genetic material. In contrast, SpeB is chromosomally encoded. Indeed, the *SpeB*

HOW SCIENTISTS DETERMINE WHICH BACTERIAL PRODUCTS ARE VIRULENCE FACTORS

Scientists use a number of different model systems (generally either cells or animals) to determine which bacterial proteins may be considered virulence factors and which ones do not appear to be involved in the pathogenesis of the bacterium. One model is blood donated by humans. Some bacteria can grow and reproduce in pure human blood. Others cannot do so; they are phagocytosed (in other words, eaten and destroyed) by killer cells in the human blood. By comparing bacteria that survive in the blood with those that do not, scientists can determine which factors may be important for bacterial survival during an actual human infection.

Another model uses pure cells grown in a petri dish. These cells can be of either human or animal origin. When bacteria are added to the cells, the bacteria can express a number of proteins. Some of these proteins may allow the bacteria to stick to the cells. This property is important during an infection; if bacteria cannot stick to cells in the throat, they will easily be washed away when the host eats or drinks, and therefore, they will be unable to start an infection.

Other model systems use living animals. The most common animal model is the mouse. Mice are fairly inexpensive to buy and house, and an investigator can choose either inbred mice (mice that have been bred with siblings, and are therefore quite similar genetically) or outbred mice (which have not been bred with relatives, and are thus more genetically vari-

gene has been found in the chromosomal DNA of every GAS isolate tested so far. This gene encodes a protease that is secreted in large quantities by many isolates. Whether this protease is a critical virulence factor of the bacteria remains a source of able). Investigators can choose mice in which human genes have been inserted (transgenic mice), or they can choose mice that lack cells that produce antibodies or other components of the immune system.

Some unique model systems have been employed in the analysis of virulence factors in *Streptococcus pyogenes*. One group of investigators used a baboon model system to study factors that led to throat colonization, and therefore, to the development of streptococcal pharyngitis. Baboons are excellent animals to study because they are very similar to humans, but they are quite expensive to work with and often very difficult to perform experiments on.

Another group of investigators used zebra fish as a model to study streptococcal virulence factors. The advantages of using these fish as models include their small size and inexpensive price. A great deal is also known about the genetics of these fish, which make it easy to analyze host-pathogen interactions. However, zebra fish are much less similar to humans than are baboons or mice.

One group of scientists has, in a way, decided to combine a mouse and a human. Debra Bessen and her colleagues at Yale University grafted human foreskin onto a SCID mouse (which is unable to reject foreign skin grafts). They then made superficial wounds on the human skin and seeded it with group A streptococci to investigate the human skin response to bacterial infection without using a human.[2]

controversy. Interestingly, SpeB is able to modify both host and bacterial proteins. Several of these bacterial proteins are those produced by genes in the Mga regulon. Release of portions of these proteins by SpeB has been hypothesized to play a role in the kidney damage seen in acute post-streptococcal glomerulonephritis.

CAPSULE

Like many bacteria, GAS can express a **capsule** (a slimy, sticky coating on the bacterium made of a chemical called hyaluronic acid). The size of the capsule has been associated with virulence in certain model systems and is a well-recognized virulence mechanism used by many human pathogens. Clinical observations have linked highly encapsulated, or **mucoid**, strains of GAS both to invasive infection and to acute rheumatic fever. Acapsular mutant strains (meaning they have no or very little capsule) of GABHS generally are not virulent in experimental models of systemic and invasive soft tissue infection.

Studies of the genetics of capsule synthesis in GAS lead to the identification of a **regulon** containing genes associated

covR/covS: SMALL CHANGES CAN MAKE A BIG DIFFERENCE

A curious phenomenon in GABHS was first noticed almost 100 years ago: passing the bacteria through human blood (or, a live animal) resulted in the recovery of bacteria which expressed much more M protein on their surfaces. Other protein expression was also affected: some proteases were turned off, for example, while other proteins were over-expressed. No one was quite sure why this happened, however, until a 2006 paper showed that a single nucleotide mutation in the *covS* gene could lead to this phenotype. Bacteria which show this phenotype have been found to be very virulent in animal models—could it be that bacteria which cause NF are these types of mutants? Additional studies are investigating this question.[3]

with capsule synthesis. Because GAS isolates can change the size of their capsule when grown under different conditions or when exposed to biological pressures in human blood, a regulator for the capsular genes was predicted (a **regulator** is a gene that controls expression of other genes). A number of groups studying capsular variants and acapsular mutants identified the two-component capsule regulatory system, *covR/covS* (called *csrR/csrS* by a different set of researchers). Mutants in this system cause enhanced virulence in a mouse model of skin and soft tissue infection. These mutants can appear spontaneously during infection and increase the severity of infection.

HEMOLYSINS: SLS AND SLO

Beta-hemolysis is one of the defining phenotypic characteristics of GAS. Hemolysis (literally, "breaking open blood cells") on blood agar plates is caused by the production of one of two hemolysins: streptolysin O (SLO; *O* for "oxygen labile," meaning that it is degraded in the presence of oxygen) or streptolysin S (SLS; *S* for "stable in the presence of oxygen"). SLO is a member of a family of pore-forming cytolysins. These are proteins that, like the complement proteins mentioned above, punch holes in other cells. They do so only where complement creates pores in bacterial cells. SLO and SLS form pores in the host's cells, and are toxic to a variety of cells. SLO is produced by almost every strain of GABHS.

SLS is produced by streptococci that are growing in the presence of human serum. It is one of the most potent known **cytotoxins** (chemicals that kill cells). Although it is stable in the presence of oxygen, it is sensitive to heat. Most isolates of GABHS produce SLS in addition to SLO, but occasionally an isolate will be found that produces only one, or, in rare instances, neither hemolysin. Interestingly, since beta-hemolysis is one of the hallmarks used to identify group A streptococci in clinical labs, isolates that produce neither hemolysin are often misidentified at first.

8

Vaccine Prospects and the Future of the Group A Streptococcus

In infectious disease research, scientists strive to better understand the pathogen to more effectively prevent and treat the disease. Information gleaned from investigations of the basic biology of an agent of disease can be used to uncover a weakness of the microbe. This knowledge will allow researchers to develop an effective treatment strategy that takes advantage of this weakness, as well as to develop strategies that will allow the host's own immune system to fight the initial onslaught of the microbe; in other words, to **vaccinate** individuals against the microbe in question. For some pathogens, effective **vaccines** were developed centuries ago. For example, the vaccine for smallpox was so effective at preventing disease that the smallpox virus, *Variola major*, for which humans are the only hosts, was eradicated from nature.

However, some pathogens continue to elude efforts to develop a safe, effective vaccine. The group A streptococcus, at the present time, is one such pathogen. Despite many decades and an enormous monetary investment, no effective, universal vaccine yet exists to protect humans against infection with GABHS. There is, however, a large amount of interest and research focused on developing such a vaccine, since it would likely save an estimated 400,000 lives that are lost each year worldwide to rheumatic fever and rheumatic heart disease alone.

26-VALENT VACCINE

As noted, much vaccine research has focused on the hypervariable M protein of GABHS. Finally, after decades of work, a vaccine just may come to fruition. Challenges to this vaccine have been discussed in the text: there are many different types of M protein, so a successful vaccine should incorporate the most common ones circulating in the population. The newly designed vaccine is referred to as "26-valent," meaning it contains 26 different types of M protein in its formulation. This will be sufficient to protect recipients against serotypes of GABHS causing 78 percent of all invasive infections, 80 percent of pharyngitis cases, and 100 percent of all "rheumatogenic" serotypes.

The vaccine formulation was first tested on rabbits, which received the vaccine and then had their immune reactions measured. The vaccine was highly effective and, importantly, it did not cause any harmful cross-reactive antibodies (which could attack the vaccine recipient's own tissues).

After animal experiments were complete, testing of the new vaccine could begin in humans, in order to determine both safety and effectiveness. Initial testing was conducted on 30 adult volunteers, which showed the vaccine to be safe and well-tolerated, without any serious side effects. A second study, with 70 volunteers, showed similar results. Both studies showed that the volunteers developed antibodies against the streptococcal M proteins included in the vaccine.

While this vaccine shows much promise, there is a downside. The M proteins chosen represent types that will be seen most commonly in developed countries, such as the United States. However, GABHS is a problem all over the world, and strains that are present in the United States may be rare in other affected countries, such as Nigeria or Nicaragua. Therefore, additional epidemiologic studies need to be carried out in order to determine the best vaccine formulation for other areas of the world, with the ultimate goal of preventing GABHS disease.[1]

VACCINE STRATEGY BASED ON THE M PROTEIN

The most promising vaccine candidates for GABHS are based on the M protein. These vaccines are generally based on the N-terminal portion of the M protein (the variable part of the protein). The N-terminal is the segment that encodes most of the determinants of serotype (the "hypervariable" portion of the protein). The goal of vaccine research in this area is to cause the body to produce an immune response against antigens of the M protein so that when the vaccinated person is infected with a strain of GABHS, the body will rapidly manufacture antibody against that portion of the M protein on the surface of the bacteria. These antibodies will then bind to the bacteria and serve as a marker to help the host's immune system destroy the invading bacterium. However, there is a limitation to this vaccination technique. Because the M protein is one bacterial factor that may contribute to the development of autoimmune sequelae, such as rheumatic fever and glomerulonephritis, using a large amount of the M protein as a vaccine may result in the development of these diseases or may make them worse in people who have previously developed them. Because there have been more than 100 serotypes of M protein described to date, a vaccine would have to include, at least, all of the most common serotypes circulating in the population. This approach is currently being tested using a vaccine containing 26 different types of M protein (see sidebar). While still experimental, if this vaccine succeeds, it will be the first licensed vaccine against GABHS in history.

A similar vaccine approach has been developed using the conserved C-terminal portion of the M protein (the portion closest to the bacterial cell), rather than the hypervariable N-terminal portion. With this approach, scientists hoped to find an **epitope** that was able to induce an antibody response against the bacteria but that did not also stimulate a cross-reactive response (in other words, it did not also cause antibodies to attack the host's own proteins). Preliminary studies suggest that such an approach is possible, and that it may be even more effective if combined with a limited number of serotypic determinants (from the variable portion of the M protein) that circulate among the population. However, adding serotypic determinants means that each vaccine would have to be manufactured with a particular region in mind. This would increase the cost. In addition, studies have shown that the most common serotype in a population can change relatively quickly (in the course of just one year). Therefore, a vaccine of this nature may have to be updated yearly, as is done with the influenza vaccine. Again, this would greatly increase the cost and limit the practicality of the vaccine.

OTHER VACCINE CANDIDATES

The C5a peptidase is another promising vaccine candidate. Studies have been carried out in mice using a portion of this protein, with an intranasal inoculation method. The vaccinated mice were found to produce antibody against the C5a peptidase and also to eliminate GABHS more quickly from their throats after they were infected than did mice that had not been vaccinated. Another advantage of using C5a peptidase instead of the M protein is that the C5a peptidase protein is highly conserved among serotypes; that is, the protein is essentially the same in all serotypes of GABHS (versus, for example, the more than 100 different varieties of the M protein). Finally, the C5a peptidase vaccine makes it harder for bacteria of different serotypes to survive on the oral mucosa (the tissue lining the mouth and throat); thus, the bacteria are less likely to remain in the mouth long enough to cause a serious infection.

Another potential vaccine candidate is the SfbI protein (fibronectin binding protein I; fibronectin is a host glycoprotein). The SfbI protein aids the bacterium in attachment to host cells, which allows for a population of bacteria to colonize the host's upper respiratory tract. Similar to the M protein, SfbI has also been shown to act as an **invasin**, allowing individual bacteria to enter human cells. It may also interfere with the immune response the host mounts against bacterial invasion. There are several advantages to producing a vaccine targeting this protein. First, the

WHY DO CHILDREN HAVE TO RECEIVE SO MANY VACCINES?

Many parents do not understand the risks and benefits of vaccines. Several stories that have appeared recently in the media suggesting a link between vaccination and diseases (such as autism) have fueled fears of vaccination in some people. However, for almost all children, these worries are unfounded.

Vaccination has effectively put an end to many of the worst diseases of childhood, such as whooping cough, measles, polio, and diphtheria. It has even led to the complete eradication of the smallpox virus from nature. Routine vaccination has significantly reduced childhood mortality rates around the world. Vaccines are held to the highest standard of safety, and are monitored constantly for any adverse side effects they might cause.

In addition, vaccination is a procedure that benefits the entire community, not just the person who gets the vaccination. This is because of an effect called herd immunity. In essence, if most of the "herd," or population, is vaccinated against a particular disease, even those who have not been vaccinated will be safer because the microbe will not be able to spread easily through a community. Therefore, one vaccinated person will help prevent disease in many others.

protein is exposed on the surface of the bacteria, which makes it an easy target for the host immune system. Second, as with C5a peptidase, the protein sequence is relatively unchanged, even in different serotypes of GABHS. In addition, SfbI is expressed by the majority of clinical isolates and does not cross-react with any known human proteins. Thus, using a vaccine against SfbI would avoid many of the problems that would occur with an M protein vaccine, including possible autoimmune reactions. Studies carried out in mice have shown that immunization with SfbI results in the production of a large amount of antibody against the protein. Studies have also shown that this vaccine protected the mice against further infection with GABHS. Additional studies are in progress.

Other bacterial proteins that have been suggested as potential vaccine candidates include the streptococcal cysteine protease SpeB. This protein has an advantage in that every isolate of GABHS found to date has been shown to possess the gene that encodes this protein. However, the protein is not always expressed (meaning that, although the bacterium may carry the gene, it may not actually produce the protein). In addition, because this is a **secreted** (released) protein rather than a surface protein, antibodies would not be directed against the bacterium, which may allow many to escape the immune response and continue to cause infection. Another candidate being explored as a possible basis for a vaccine is the group A carbohydrate. A combination vaccine that consists of several of these potential candidates is another, and perhaps the best, alternative.

CONCLUSION

The group A streptococcus was one of our first identified bacterial nemeses. Despite over 100 years of investigation into this organism, we still know comparatively little about how it causes human disease, and why the epidemiology of these diseases has changed over the decades. Additionally, while many infectious diseases have been eradicated (or nearly so) due to successful vaccination campaigns, we still lack a safe and effective vaccine against *Streptococcus pyogenes*. What we do know is that the group A streptococcus has long been a scourge of humanity, whether it is due to its manifestation in diseases such as childbed fever, scarlet fever, necrotizing fasciitis, or run-of-the-mill strep throat, or due to post-infectious sequelae such as rheumatic heart disease or glomerulonephritis. While the successful development of a vaccine may minimize streptococcal disease, it remains likely that the group A streptococcus will be with humanity for a long time to come.

Notes

Chapter 2

1. E. M. O'Hern, "Rebecca Craighill Lancefield, Pioneer Microbiologist," *ASM News* 41 (1975): 805–810.
2. J. R. Casey and M. E. Pichichero, "The Evidence Base for Cephalosporin Superiority over Penicillin in Streptococcal Pharyngitis," *Diagnostic Microbiology and Infectous Disease* 57 (3 Suppl): 39S–45S.
3. A. G. Michos et al., "Macrolide Resistance in Streptococcus pyogenes: Prevalence, Resistance Determinants, and emm Types," *Diagnostic Microbiology and Infectious Disease* 64, no. 3 (July 2009): 295–9.

Chapter 3

1. G. Falkenhorst et al., "Outbreak of Group A Streptococcal Throat Infection: Don't Forget to Ask About Food," *Epidemiology and Infection* 136 (2008): 1165–71.

Chapter 5

1. L. M. Young and C. S. Price, "Community-acquired Methicillin-resistant Staphylococcus aureus Emerging as an Important Cause of Necrotizing Fasciitis," *Surgical Infections* 9, no. 4 (August 2008): 469–74.
2. R. H. Baevsky, J. T. Ishida, and S. A. Lieberman, "Group A Beta-hemolytic Streptococcal Glossal Necrotizing Myositis—Case Report and Review," *Medscape General Medicine* 7, no. 2 (June 30, 2005): 8.

Chapter 7

1. M. D. P. Boyle, "Variation of Multifunctional Surface Binding Proteins—A Virulence Strategy for Group A Streptococci?" *Journal of Theoretical Biology* 173 (1995): 415–426; M. G. Caparon and J. R. Scott, "Identification of a Gene that Regulates Expression of M Protein, the Major Virulence Determinant of Group A Streptococci," *Proceedings of the National Academy of Sciences* 84 (1987): 8677–8681; M. W. Cunningham, "Pathogenesis of Group A Streptococcal Infections," *Clinical Microbiology Reviews* 13 (2000): 470–511; and V. A. Fischetti, "Surface Proteins on Gram-positive Bacteria," *Gram-Positive Pathogens*, eds. V. A. Fischetti et al. (Washington, D.C.: American Society for Microbiology, 2000), 11–24.
2. C. D. Ashbaugh et al., "Bacterial Determinants of Persistent Throat Colonization and the Associated Immune Response in a Primate Model of Human Group A Streptococcal Pharyngeal Infection," *Current Microbiology* 2 (2000): 283–292; M. N. Neely, J. D. Pfeifer, and M. G. Caparon, "Streptococcus-zebrafish Model of Bacterial Pathogenesis," *Infection and Immunity* 70 (2002): 3904–3914; and D. A. Scaramuzzino, J. M. Niff, and D. E. Bessen, "Humanized In Vivo Model for Streptococcal Impetigo," *Infection and Immunity* 68 (2000): 2880–2887.
3. P. Sumby et al., "Genome-wide Analysis of Group A Streptococci Reveals a Mutation that Modulates Global Phenotype and Disease Specificity" *PLoS Pathogens* 2, no. 1 (January 2006): e5.

Chapter 8

1. J. B. Dale, "Current Status of Group A Streptococcal Vaccine Development," *Advances in Experimental Medicine and Biology* 609 (2008): 53–63.

acute post-streptococcal glomerulonephritis—A postinfection consequence affecting the kidneys that may follow *S. pyogenes* infection, characterized by inflammatory changes in glomeruli capillaries. *See also* **glomerulonephritis.**

alleles—Different forms of similar genes.

amino acids—The building blocks that make up proteins.

antibiotic resistance—The phenomenon in which bacteria acquire genes that allow them to survive in the presence of antibacterial drugs.

antibodies—Proteins present in the blood that recognize and bind to specific portions of bacterial proteins.

antigen—Portion of a protein that a specific bacterium produces; antigens elicit an immune response.

antigen-antibody complex—Associations between portions of the bacterial protein (antigens) and the host's defense molecules (antibodies).

antigenic cross-reaction—The phenomenon that occurs when an antibody, generated toward a microbial protein, instead targets a host protein with a similar structure.

antiphagocytic protein—A protein that can prevent a host's phagocytes from effectively destroying invading antigens.

antisera—Serums that contain specific antibodies.

aseptic—Sterile.

asymptomatic carrier—A person who shows no signs of illness, yet is able to transmit disease to others.

autoimmune disease—Illness that results when the body's immune system attacks host cells rather than invading microbes.

bacteriophage—Virus that infects bacteria; in some cases, it becomes part of the bacteria's genome.

B cells—Cells of the host's immune system that produce antibodies.

blood agar plate—Growth medium used for culture of group A streptococci; it consists of sheep red blood cells in an agar base.

capsule—An extracellular protective coating produced by some isolates of group A streptococci.

Centers for Disease Control and Prevention (CDC)—Based in Atlanta, Georgia, the premier institution for infectious disease research in the United States.

C5a peptidase—A protein that cuts up and destroys the host complement protein C5a; it is encoded by a streptococcal gene named *scpA*.

ciliated cells—Cells with a tail-like structure that help move bacteria out of the lungs.

coccus—Sphere-shaped bacterium.

complement—A set of plasma proteins that act together to attack bacterial pathogens, which they destroy by creating a hole in the bacterial cell wall.

contagious—Capable of transmitting a disease to others.

cytokines—Host proteins that play an important role in controlling the reactions of the host immune system.

cytotoxin—A chemical that kills cells.

edema—Localized swelling.

efficacy—Effectiveness; the ability of a drug to cure or control an illness.

***emm* gene superfamily**—A series of genes that arose by duplication and encode for proteins with similar, but distinct, functions. Genes in this group include *emm, mrp,* and *enn.*

encephalitis—Inflammation of the brain.

endemic—A disease that is common in a population.

epidemiology—The study of disease patterns.

epitope—Specific segments of protein that elicit an immune response.

erythema—Feeling of warmth in a diseased area; often accompanies edema.

erythromycin—A common antibiotic used to treat infections caused by group A streptococci.

etiology—In infectious disease studies, the root cause of the disease.

extracellular pathogen—A pathogen that lives outside of the host's cells.

fascia—The tissue underlying the skin.

fatality rate—Measurement of the number of persons who, upon contracting a particular disease, will die from it. *See also* **mortality.**

febris scarlatina—Original Latin name given to the disease scarlet fever by the British physician Thomas Sydenham.

genotype—The genetic makeup of an organism.

germ theory of disease—Scientific theory that describes how microorganisms, including bacteria, viruses, fungi, and parasites, cause contagious diseases.

glomeruli—The filtering tubules that make up the kidneys.

glomerulonephritis—A kidney disease characterized by inflammatory changes in glomeruli capillaries. See also **acute post-streptococcal glomerulonephritis.**

gram-positive—Bacteria that, when stained by the Gram method, appear purple. Gram-negative bacteria will appear pink.

Gram stain—Method used to differentiate bacteria based on characteristics of the bacterial cell wall. Gram-negative bacteria will appear pink, while gram-positive bacteria will appear purple.

hemolysin—A protein produced by most isolates of *S. pyogenes* that lyses (breaks open) red blood cells.

hemolytic—Capable of lysing (breaking open) red blood cells.

healthy carrier—*See* **asymptomatic carrier.**

herd immunity—The condition that arises when many members of a population are vaccinated against a disease and, in becoming immune, help prevent even those who are not vaccinated from becoming ill.

humors—An ancient way of characterizing the fluids in the body; the four humors were blood, black bile, yellow bile, and phlegm; an "imbalance" of these fluids was considered to be the cause of disease.

immune—Unable to be reinfected by a particular type of organism.

immune system—The host's main defense against microbial invaders, consisting of antibodies.

impetigo—A skin infection caused by group A streptococci, which generally begins as small blisters. When these blisters burst, reddish patches of skin are revealed, which may ooze fluid. A yellowish crust will form as the infection heals.

incidence—The number of new cases of disease in a population within a given period.

incubation period—The amount of time it takes from the initial exposure to the infectious agent to the development of disease.

intracellular pathogen—A pathogen that lives within the host's cells.

intranasal—Inside the nose; a way of administering doses of vaccines or bacteria to experimental animals.

intravenous—Drugs that are administered directly into the bloodstream.

invasin—A protein that facilitates bacterial invasion of host cells.

invasive disease—A disease that spreads throughout the body, generally via the blood. Invasive diseases generally have a significantly higher fatality rate than **superficial diseases**.

in vitro—Outside of a living system.

isolate—An individual isolation of bacteria from an infected host.

localized—Confined to a particular (generally small) area of the host's body, without spreading to other areas.

lochia—Vaginal discharge that occurs in the weeks following childbirth.

major histocompatibility complex (MHC)—A set of proteins encoded by host genes that allow the host's immune system to recognize specific pathogens. Certain types of these genes are more frequently associated with autoimmune diseases, such as rheumatic fever.

meningitis—Inflammation of the meninges, the membranes surrounding the brain and spinal cord.

Mga regulon—Genes present in the group A streptococcus whose expression is controlled by the expression of a common gene, termed *mga*. Genes in this regulon include *emm, mrp, enn, scpA,* and *sic*.

miasmas—Literally, "bad airs" that were thought to be a cause of disease prior to the development of the germ theory of disease.

mortality—See **fatality rate.**

M protein—Protein encoded by the *emm* gene; an antiphagocytic surface protein present on the surface of group A streptococci. Characteristics of this protein are responsible for the serotyping scheme developed by Rebecca Lancefield.

mucoid—Isolates of group A streptococci producing large amounts of capsule.

mucous membranes—The inner lining of the mouth and nasal passages, or any lining containing cells that secrete mucus.

mucus—A slimy secretion of cells of the mucous membranes, composed of various salts, cells, and chemicals.

myosin—A protein that makes up part of the structure of muscle, including the heart.

myositis—A very rare invasive disease caused by group A streptococci, in which bacteria invade and destroy the muscle of the heart.

nasopharyngeal passages—Passageways connecting the nose and the throat.

necrosis—Death of body tissue.

necrotizing fasciitis (NF)—A disease caused by group A streptococci, also known as "flesh-eating disease." NF is characterized by localized swelling and pain, often following a scratch or bruise in the area. This proceeds to cause extreme tissue damage, resulting in removal of the tissue in the area, and possibly death.

nephritogenic—Strain of group A streptococci that is capable of causing glomerulonephritis.

normal flora—Bacteria that coexist with the host, usually in a mutually beneficial relationship. Normal flora do not cause disease under most circumstances.

opacity factor—A protein produced by some isolates of group A streptococci. When present, it causes serum to become opaque.

PANDAS—Pediatric autoimmune neuropsychiatric disorders associated with streptococcal infections. Refers to a group of diseases that are thought to be autoimmune in nature, and have been linked to infection by group A streptococci.

pathogenic—Causing disease in a host.

pathology—Destruction of body tissue caused by disease.

petri dish—A plastic container used to grow cells. The dish may be filled with agar, to provide a solid nutrient base on which bacteria can grow; or cells (such as human tissue cells) may be seeded directly onto the dish and bathed in a nutrient media.

phagocyte—Cell of the host immune system that seeks out and destroys invading pathogens.

phagocytosis—The process by which a white blood cell engulfs and destroys a foreign organism, such as a bacterium or virus.

pharyngitis—Painful inflammation of the throat. When caused by the group A streptococcus, symptoms also include chills, fever, body aches, and spots of pus on the tonsils (see also **tonsillopharyngitis**).

phenotype—Physical characteristics of an organism.

postinfection sequelae—Diseases, generally autoimmune in nature, that occur following clearance of the original pathogen. Singular of *sequelae* is *sequel.*

postmortem—Occurring after death.

predispose—Make one more vulnerable.

protease—A protein that cleaves other proteins.

protective immunity—Previous exposure to the pathogen, which will allow for a quicker antibody response the second time the pathogen is encountered, thereby protecting the host from reinfection.

puerperal fever—Also known as "childbed fever;" a streptococcal infection of the blood that may occur following childbirth.

pus—Material consisting of white blood cells and extracellular fluid that comes from a wound.

reemerging pathogen—A classification given to an established human pathogen that has recently increased in virulence.

regulator—A gene whose product controls the expression of other genes.

regulon—Two or more separate genes that work together because of the influence of another molecule, or regulator.

resistance—See **antibiotic resistance**.

rheumatagenic—Strains of group A streptococci that are capable of causing rheumatic fever.

rheumatic fever—An autoimmune sequel to infection with certain serotypes of group A streptococci. Symptoms include fever and arthritis in the joints; rheumatic fever can eventually cause damage to the heart.

rheumatic heart disease—Also known as **rheumatic carditis**, a common consequence of rheumatic fever, due to damage of the heart valves. Rheumatic heart disease is the leading cause of death from cardiac disease among young people in developing countries.

risk factor—A factor that, when present, increases the likelihood of developing a particular disease.

scabies—A skin rash caused by mites.

scarlet fever—A disease that may occur following a group A streptococcal throat infection. The disease is characterized by a red rash and high fever, and is thought to be due to the production of toxins by the infecting bacteria.

secreted—A protein that is released extracellularly, away from the cell that produced it.

septicemia—Presence of bacteria in the bloodstream.

serotype—A specific reaction of antibodies to certain properties of a bacterium.

sequence—As a noun, *sequence* refers to the string of base pairs that make up an organism's DNA. As a verb, it refers to the active process of determining the order of these base pairs in a portion of the organism's DNA.

shock—A decrease in blood pressure or volume, resulting in a lack of blood flow to the organs. May result in death.

strain—Bacteria that share the same genotype or phenotype; clones.

streptococcal pyrogenic exotoxins (SPEs)—Toxins produced by some isolates of group A streptococci, which cause may cause rash and/or shock.

streptococcal toxic shock syndrome (STSS)—Streptococcal disease characterized by the rapid onset of severe pain and fever; a rash may also be present. STSS may rapidly lead to death due to multiple organ failure.

subcutaneous—Beneath the skin.

subdermal—Beneath the dermis, a lower layer of the skin.

sulfonamides—A group of antibiotics.

superantigen—A protein that is capable of stimulating the immune system, causing it to behave abnormally.

superficial disease—Generally a nonlethal disease. Infection is usually confined to a small area of the patient's body and does not spread via the bloodstream.

Sydenham chorea—A neurological sequel of infection with the group A streptococcus, characterized by jerky, uncontrollable movements, either of the face or of the arms and legs.

tachycardia—A very rapid heartbeat.

tics—Spasmodic involuntary muscular contractions most commonly involving the face, mouth, eyes, head, neck, or shoulder muscles.

tonsillopharyngitis—*See* **pharyngitis**.

toxic shock syndrome (TSS)—An invasive disease caused by a bacterium called *Staphylococcus aureus*. Many cases of this disease were seen in women in the late 1970s and were associated with the use of tampons. Clinical symptoms are similar to those seen in STSS.

toxins—Poisons that may be produced by isolates of bacteria.

vaccinate—To give a vaccine, in order to make someone immune to a particular pathogen or disease.

vaccines—Suspensions of either dead or attenuated (weakened) pathogen, or products produced by a pathogen, designed to cause immunity to the pathogen in the host.

virulence—The severity of clinical illness resulting from infection.

virulence factor—Proteins expressed by bacteria that contribute to their ability to cause a clinical infection in the host.

Adam, D. "Introduction to Group A Streptococcal Treatment." *Journal of Antimicrobial Chemotherapy* 45 (2000): 1–2.

Adriaanse, A. H., M. Pel, and O. P. Bleker. "Semmelweis: The Combat Against Puerperal Fever." *European Journal of Obstetrics & Gynecology and Reproductive Biology* 90, no. 2 (2000): 153–158.

Androulla, Efstratiou. "Group A Streptococci in the 1990s." *Journal of Antimicrobial Chemotherapy* 45 (2000): 3–12.

Bessen, D. E. "Genetics of Childhood Disorders: XXXII. Autoimmune Disorders, Part 5: Streptococcal Infection and Autoimmunity, an Epidemiological Perspective." *Journal of the American Academy of Child and Adolescent Psychiatry* 40, no. 11 (2001): 1346–1348.

Betschel, S. D., S. M. Borgia, N. L. Barg, D. E. Low, and J. C. DeAzavedo. "Reduced Virulence of Group A Streptococcal Tn916 Mutants That Do Not Produce Streptolysin S." *Infection and Immunity* 66 (1998): 1671–1679.

Bisno, A. L., M. A. Gerber, J. M. Gwaltney, E. L. Kaplan, and R. H. Schwartz. "Practice Guidelines for the Diagnosis and Management of Group A Streptococcal Pharyngitis." *Clinical Infectious Diseases* 35 (2000): 113–125.

Boyle, M.D.P. "Variation of Multifunctional Surface Binding Proteins — A Virulence Strategy for Group A Streptococci?" *Journal of Theoretical Biology* 173, no. 4 (1995): 415–426.

Caparon, M. G., and J. R. Scott. "Identification of a Gene that Regulates Expression of M Protein, the Major Virulence Determinant of Group A Streptococci." *Proceedings of the National Academy of Sciences USA* 84 (1987): 8677–8681.

Chapin, K. C., P. Blake, and C. D. Wilson. "Performance Characteristics and Utilization of Rapid Antigen Test, DNA Probe, and Culture for Detection of Group A Streptococci in an Acute Care Clinic." *Journal of Clinical Microbiology* 40 (2002): 4207–4210.

Chaussee, M. S., G. L. Sylva, D. E. Sturdevant, L. M. Smoot, M. R. Grahamp, R. O. Watson, and J. M. Musser. "Rgg Influences the Expression of Multiple Regulatory Loci to Coregulate Virulence Factor Expression in *Streptococcus Pyogenes.*" *Infection and Immunity* 70 (2002): 762–770.

Cleary, P. P., J. Handley, A. N. Suvorov, A. Podbielski, and P. Ferrieri. "Similarity Between the Group B and A Streptococcal C5a Peptidase Genes." *Infection and Immunity* 60 (1992): 4239–4244.

Couser, W. G. "Glomerulonephritis." *Lancet* 353, no. 9163 (1999): 1509–1515.

Currie, B. J., and J. R. Carapetis. "Skin Infections and Infestations in Aboriginal Communities in Northern Austrialia." *Australasian Journal of Dermatology* 41 (2000): 139–145.

Debré, Patrice. *Louis Pasteur.* Baltimore: Johns Hopkins University Press, 2000.

Engleberg, N. C., A. Heath, A. Miller, C. Rivera, and V. J. DiRita. "Spontaneous Mutations in the CsrRS Two-component Regulatory System of *Streptococcus Pyogenes* Result in Enhanced Virulence in a Murine Model of Skin and Soft Tissue Infection." *Journal of Infectious Diseases* 183 (2001): 1043–1054.

Espinosa de los Monteros, L. E., I. M. Bustos, L. V. Flores, and C. Avila-Figueroa. "Outbreak of Scarlet Fever Caused by an Erythromycin-resistant Streptococcus Pyogenes emm22 Genotype Strain in a Day-care Center." *Pediatric Infectious Disease Journal* 20, no. 8 (2001): 807–809.

Fischetti, V. A. "Surface Proteins on Gram-positive Bacteria." *Gram-Positive Pathogens*, eds. V. A. Fischetti, R. P. Novick, J. J. Ferretti, D. A. Portnoy, and J. I. Rood. Washington, D.C.: American Society for Microbiology, 2000, pp. 11–24.

Frick, I. M., M. Morgelin, and L. Bjorck. "Virulent Aggregates of Streptococcus Pyogenes are Generated by Homophilic Protein-protein Interactions." *Molecular Microbiology* 37 (2000): 1232–1247.

Garrett, Laurie. *The Coming Plague.* New York: Penguin Books, 1995.

Gerber, M. A. "Antibiotic resistance: relationship to persistence of group A streptococci in the upper respiratory tract." *Pediatrics* 97 (1996): 971–975.

Good, M. F. "Progress toward Developing a Vaccine for Group A Streptococcus Based on the M Protein." *Internal Medicine Journal* 32 (2002): 132–133.

Haukness, H. A., R. R. Tanz, R. B. Thomson, Jr., D. K. Pierry, E. L. Kaplan, B. Beall, D. Johnson, N. P. Hoe, J. M. Musser, and S. T. Shulman. "The Heterogeneity of Endemic Community Pediatric Group A Streptococcal Pharyngeal Isolates and Their Relationship to Invasive Isolates." *Journal of Infectious Diseases* 185 (2002): 915–920.

Hilario, M., and M. Terreri. "Rheumatic Fever and Post-streptococcal Arthritis." *Best Practice and Research Clinical Rheumatology* 16, no. 3 (2002): 481–494.

Hoe, N. P., R. M. Ireland, F. R. DeLeo, B. B. Gowen, D. W. Dorward, J. M. Voyich, M. Liu, E. H. Burns, D. M. Culnan, A. Bretscher, and J. M. Musser. "Insight into the Molecular Basis of Pathogen Abundance: Group A Streptococcus Inhibitor of Complement Inhibits Bacterial Adherence and Internalization into Human Cells." *Proceedings of the National Academy of Sciences USA* 99 (2002): 7646–7651.

Ji, Y., B. Carlson, A. Kondagunta, and P. P. Cleary. "Intranasal Immunization with C5a Peptidase Prevents Nasopharyngeal Colonization of Mice by the Group A Streptococcus." *Infection and Immunity* 65 (1997): 2080–2087.

Kapur, V., J. Maffei, G. Greer, G. Adams, J. M. Musser. "Vaccination with Streptococcal Extracellular Cysteine Protease (interleukin-1 convertase) Protects Mice against Challenge with Heterologous Group A Streptococci." *Microbial Pathogenesis* 16, no. 6 (1994): 443–450.

Karlen, A. *Man and Microbes*. New York: Simon & Schuster, 1995.

Katz, A. R., and D. M. Morens. "Severe Streptococcal Infections in Historical Perspective." *Clinical Infectious Disease* 14 (1992): 298–307.

Low, D. E., B. Schwartz, and A. McGeer. "The Reemergence of Severe Group A Streptococcal Disease: An Evolutionary Perspective." *Emerging Infections* Set 1, eds. W. M. Scheld, D. Armstrong, and J. M Hughes. Washington, D.C.: ASM Press, 1998.

Lukomski, S., N. P. Hoe, I. Abdi, J. Rurangirwa, P. Kordari, M. Liu, S. J. Dou, G. G. Adams, and J. M. Musser. "Nonpolar Inactivation of the Hypervariable Streptococcal Inhibitor of Complement Gene (*sic*) in Serotype M1 *Streptococcus Pyogenes* Significantly Decreases Mouse Mucosal Colonization." *Infection and Immunity* 68 (2000): 535–542.

McNeil, William. *Plagues and Peoples*. New York: Doubleday, 1998.

Nordstrand, A., M. Norgren, and S. E. Holm. "Pathogenic Mechanism of Acute Post-Streptococcal Glomerulonephritis." *Scandanavian Journal of Infectious Disease* 31 (1999): 523–537.

O'Brien, K. L., et al. "Epidemiology of Invasive Group a Streptococcus Disease in the United States, 1995–1999." *Clinical Infectious Diseases* 35 (2002): 268–276.

O'Hern, E. M. "Rebecca Craighill Lancefield, Pioneer Microbiologist." *ASM News* 41 (1975): 805–810.

Oliver, C. "Rheumatic Fever—Is It Still a Problem?" *Journal of Antimicrobial Chemotherapy* 45 (2000): 13–21.

Perea-Mejia, L. M., A. E. Inzunza-Montiel, and A. Cravioto. "Molecular Characterization of Group A Streptococcus Strains Isolated during a Scarlet Fever Outbreak." *Journal of Clinical Microbiology* 40 (2002): 278–280.

Podbielski, A., N. Schnitzler, P. Behys, and M.D.P. Boyle. "M-related Protein (Mrp) Contributes to Group A Streptococcal Resistance to Phagocytosis by Human Granulocytes." *Molecular Microbiology* 19 (1996): 429–441.

Roemmele, J. A., and Bardorf, D. *Surviving the "Flesh-Eating Bacteria."* New York: Avery, 2000.

Salyers, A., and D. Whitt. *Bacterial Pathogenesis: A Molecular Approach.* Washington, D.C.: ASM Press, 1994.

Saouda, M., W. Wu, P. Conran, and M.D.P. Boyle. "Streptococcal Pyrogenic Exotoxin B Enhances Tissue Damage Initiated by Other *Streptococcus Pyogenes* Products." *Journal of Infectious Diseases* 184 (2001): 723–731.

Sarkissian, A., M. Papazian, G. Azatian, N. Arikiants, A. Babloyan, and E. Leumann. "An Epidemic of Acute Postinfectious Glomerulonephritis in Armenia." *Archives of Disease in Childhood* 77 (1997): 342–344.

Schulze, K., E. Medina, G. S. Chhatwal, C. A.Guzman. "Stimulation of Long-lasting Protection against *Streptococcus Pyogenes* after Intranasal Vaccination with non Adjuvanted Fibronectin-binding Domain of the SfbI Protein." *Vaccine* 16, no. 21 (2003): 1958–1964.

Smith, T. C., D. D. Sledjeski, and M.D.P. Boyle. "Regulation of Protein H expression in M1 Serotype Isolates of *Streptococcus Pyogenes.*" *FEMS Microbiology Letters* 219, no. 1 (2003): 9–15.

Stevens, D. L. "Invasive Streptococcal Infections." *Journal of Infection and Chemotherapy* 7 (2001): 69–80.

———. "Streptococcal toxic-shock syndrome: Spectrum of Disease, Pathogenesis, and New Concepts in Treatment." *Emerging Infectious Diseases* 1 (1995): 69–78.

Strollerman, G. H. "Changing Streptococci and Prospects for the Global Eradication of Rheumatic Fever." *Perspectives in Biology and Medicine* 40 (1996): 165–189.

———. "Rheumatic Fever in the 21st Century." *Clinical Infectious Diseases* 33 (2001): 806–814.

Swedo, S. E. "Pediatric Autoimmune Neuropsychiatric Disorders Associated with Streptococcal Infections (PANDAS)." *Molecular Psychiatry* 7 (2002): S24–S25.

Vitali, L. A., C. Zampaloni, M. Prenna, and S. Ripa. "PCR M Typing: A New Method for Rapid Typing of Group A Streptococci." *Journal of Clinical Microbiology* 40 (2002): 679–681.

Wessels, M. R., J. B. Goldberg, E. A. Moses, and T. J. DiCesare. "Effects on virulence of mutations in a locus essential for hyaluronic acid capsule expression in group A streptococci." *Infection and Immunity* 62 (1994): 433–441.

Williams, Margery. *The Velveteen Rabbit.* Philadelphia: Running Press, 1981.

Further Resources

Articles

Cunningham, M. W. "Pathogenesis of Group A Streptococcal Infections." *Clinical Microbiology Reviews* 13 (2000): 470–511.

Kotb, M., A. Norrby-Teglund, A. McGeer, H. El-Sherbini, M. T. Dorak, A. Khurshid, K. Green, J. Peeples, J. Wade, G. Thomson, B. Schwartz, D. E. Low. "An Immunogenetic and Molecular Basis for Differences in Outcomes of Invasive Group A Streptococcal Infections." *Nature Medicine* 8 (2002): 1398–1404.

Web Sites

American Heart Association
http://www.americanheart.org

American Society for Microbiology
http://www.asmusa.org

Centers for Disease Control and Prevention
http://www.cdc.gov

KidsHealth
http://www.kidshealth.org

National Necrotizing Fasciitis Foundation
http://www.nnff.org

World Health Organization
http://www.who.int

Index

role in lives of prominent people,
42–43
and SpeA superantigen, 79
symptoms, 35–36, 40
Schick, Béla, 57
Schottmuller, Hugo, 57
scpA (streptococcal C5a peptidase),
77–78
scpA genes
and class II M proteins, 75
and streptococcal C5a peptidase, 78
secondary bacterial infections, 40
secreted protein
defined, 97
Sic as, 78
and SpeB protein-based vaccine,
89
Semmelweis, Ignaz, *12, 12*–14
septicemia, 14, 97
septic shock, 40
sequences, 25, 97
serotypes
and APSGN, 62
defined, 97
and *emm* genes, 73
and M proteins, 23–25, 72–76
and M protein vaccine strategy, 86,
87
and rheumatic fever, 58, 60
and Sic, 78
and streptococcal C5a peptidase, 78
SfbI protein-based vaccine, 87–89
shock, 40, 97. *See also* streptococcal
toxic shock syndrome
Sic (streptococcal inhibitor of
complement-mediated lysis),
78–79
Sic gene, 78
skin infections, 61, 62
SLO (streptolysin O), 83
SLS (streptolysin S), 83
smallpox, 88
sof gene, 75
SpeA superantigens, 79

Speb gene, 79–80
SpeB protein-based vaccine, 89
SpeB superantigens, 79–82
SPEs (streptococcal pyrogenic
exotoxins), 40, 97
Staphylococcus aureus
and impetigo, 31
and MRSA, 52
and toxic shock syndrome, 48–50,
52
strain, 22, 97
strep throat. *See* streptococcal pharyngitis
streptococcal bacteremia. *See* bacteremia
streptococcal C5a peptidase *(scpA),*
77–78
streptococcal gangrene. *See* necrotizing fasciitis
streptococcal inhibitor of complement-mediated lysis (Sic), 78–79
streptococcal myositis, 54
streptococcal pharyngitis, 27–31, *29,*
57
streptococcal pyrogenic exotoxins
(SPEs), 40, 97
streptococcal toxic shock syndrome
(STSS)
characteristics of, 16–17
cytokines and, 79
defined, 97
and GABHS, 8
outbreaks in 1980s, 50–51
Streptococcus pyogenes. See also group
A beta-hemolytic streptococcus
coining of name, 18
discovery of, 12–16
and model systems for virulence
factors, 81
streptolysin O (SLO), 83
streptolysin S (SLS), 83
STSS. *See* streptococcal toxic shock
syndrome
subcutaneous tissue, 51–52, 98

About the Author

Tara C. Smith obtained her B.S. in Biology from Yale University in New Haven, Connecticut, where she carried out research on the molecular epidemiology of *Streptococcus pyogenes*. In 2002, she earned her Ph.D. at the Medical College of Ohio in Toledo, Ohio, under the tutelage of Dr. Michael Boyle and Dr. Darren Sledjeski. Her doctoral studies focused on group A streptococci, specifically virulence factor regulation in response to biological selection pressures. She has published articles in scientific journals as a result of this research. Currently, Dr. Smith is an Assistant Professor of Infectious Disease Epidemiology at the University of Iowa, and Deputy Director of the Center for Emerging Infectious Diseases. Her research centers on zoonotic diseases (diseases transmitted between humans and animals), including *Staphylococcus aureus* and *Streptococcus suis*. She resides in Iowa with her two children.

About the Consulting Editor

Hilary Babcock, M.D., M.P.H., is an assistant professor of medicine at Washington University School of Medicine and the medical director of occupational health for Barnes-Jewish Hospital and St. Louis Children's Hospital. She received her undergraduate degree from Brown University and her M.D. from the University of Texas Southwestern Medical Center at Dallas. After completing her residency, chief residency, and Infectious Disease fellowship at Barnes-Jewish Hospital, she joined the faculty of the Infectious Disease division. She completed an M.P.H. in Public Health from St. Louis University School of Public Health in 2006. She has lectured, taught, and written extensively about infectious diseases, their treatment, and their prevention. She is a member of numerous medical associations and is board certified in infectious disease. She lives in St. Louis, Missouri.